home health massage

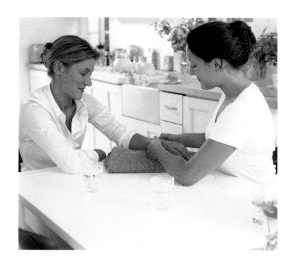

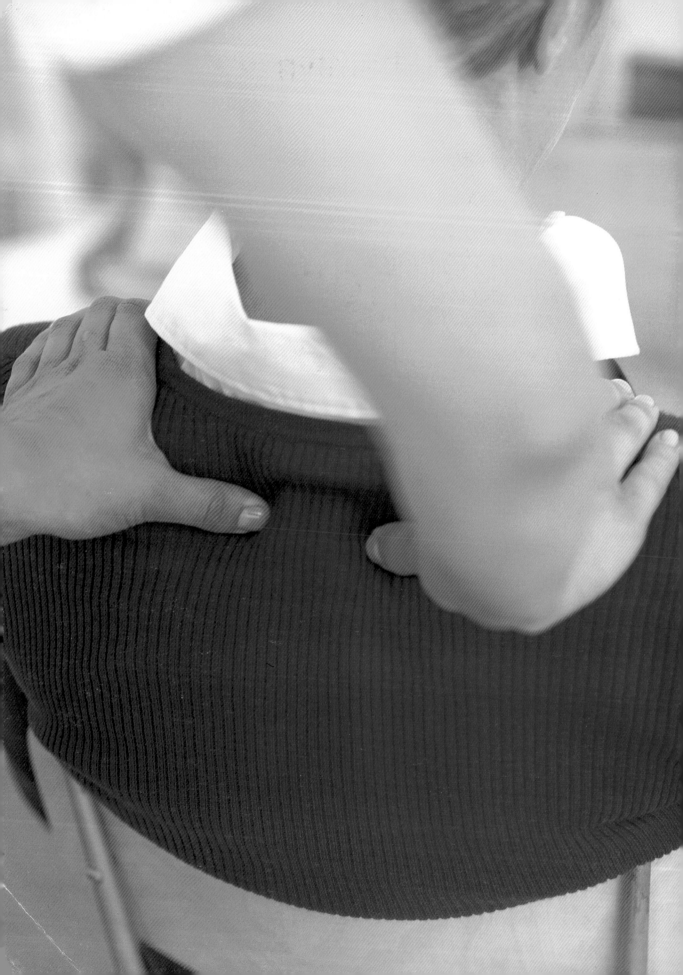

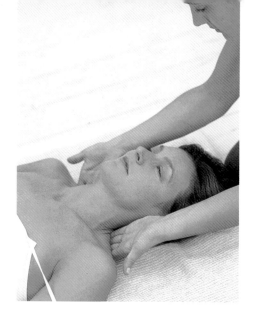

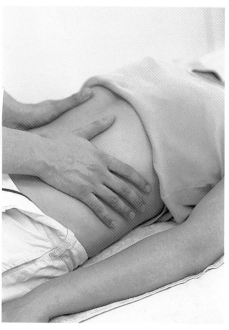

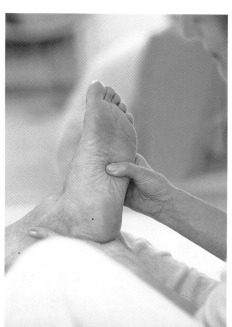

hamlyn

home
health
massage

wendy
kavanagh

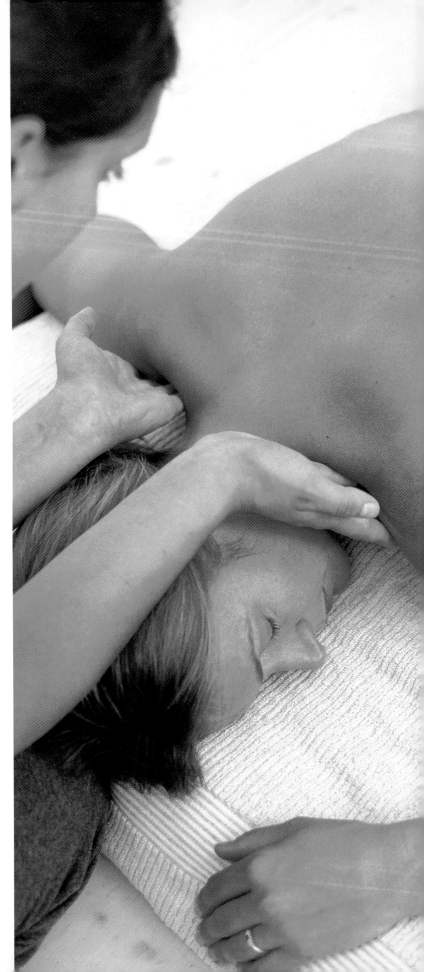

First published in Great Britain in 2002
by Hamlyn, a division of
Octopus Publishing Group Ltd
2–4 Heron Quays, London E14 4JP

Distributed in the United States and Canada by
Sterling Publishing Co., Inc.
387 Park Avenue South, New York,
NY 10016-8810

ISBN 0 600 60509 4

A CIP catalogue record for this book is available
from the British Library

Printed and bound in China

10 9 8 7 6 5 4 3 2 1

**It is advisable to check with your doctor
before embarking on any massage
programme.** Home Health Massage should
not be considered a replacement for
professional medical treatment; a physician
should be consulted in all matters relating to
health and particularly in respect of
pregnancy and any symptoms which may
require diagnosis or medical attention.While
the advice and information in this book is
believed to be accurate and the step-by-
step instructions have been devised to avoid
strain, the publisher cannot accept legal
responsibility for any injury or illness
sustained while following the massages.

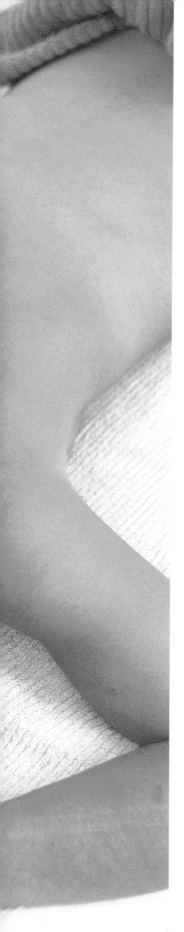

Contents

Introduction

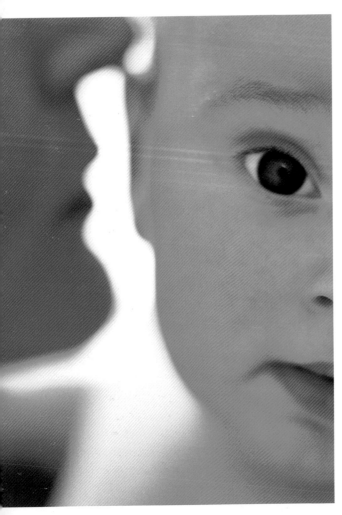

One definition of touch is 'to make physical contact, to affect emotionally' and, interestingly, it is the very first sense we develop. By the sixth week of pregnancy the tactile sense has already started to evolve in the foetus and to create the basis for all our other tools of communication. As newborns we touch to survive, and the quality of the touch we receive as we grow up will determine our levels of self-esteem, our ability to form lasting relationships with others and our capacity to be comfortable with ourselves, both physically and mentally.

Touching for Health and Happiness

Touch in the form of massage has been practised for thousands of years and its effects have been well documented, telling us clearly that massage is good for us – regular practice means we become calmer, healthier and happier. So how does it work?

Under the skin, massage causes complex processes to start up: hormones and 'signal substances' transmit messages to the brain and back again, some stimulating and others calming. Touch is known to increase the level of oxytocin, the hormone that makes us stop what we are doing and relax, which in our fast-paced modern lives is a necessary catalyst to restoring balance in our physical, emotional and spiritual well-being.

As the saying goes: 'money doesn't buy health or happiness.' It is the aim of this book to demonstrate how massage can be used as a home health programme for all the family, the only costs being gifts of time and instinctive touch. As in many traditional cultures, you can now make massage an integral part of your family life.

WHY MASSAGE?

- The word 'massage' comes from the Greek *massein*, 'to knead', which is descriptive of a technique that forms part of massage as it is practised today.
- 'Therapeutic touch' also comes from the Greek *therapeutikos*, relating to the effect of medical treatment.
- Until the 19th century, instead of 'massage' Americans used the term *frictio*, from the Latin meaning 'rubbing' or 'friction'.
- In India massage was known as *shampooing*, in China as *cong-fou* and Japan as *ambouk*.
- The term 'Swedish massage' is often used today, referring to Per Henrik Ling, a native of Sweden who was an early pioneer of the massage movement in the Western world (see opposite).

How Did it all Begin?

Massage in some form is the earliest known therapeutic art, with an extensive and well-documented history. Before that we can only speculate that there was an equally strong instinct to stroke or touch the human body.

25th century BC: The medical text known as the *Nei Ching* contains the earliest Chinese references.

24th century: Wall paintings depict massage and reflexology on a physician's tomb in Saqqara. References by Egyptian, Persian and Japanese physicians to the benefits and usefulness of massage appear.

19th century: The books of the Indian *Ayur Veda* refer to massage (as 'rubbing' and 'shampooing') as a means of helping the body to heal itself.

5th century: Herodicus and his pupil Hippocrates claim they can improve muscle tone and joint function by 'rubbing'; they also pronounce that strokes should be carried out in a direction towards the heart, as advocated today. Homer's *Odyssey* describes how exhausted war heroes are treated to oil rubdowns for restorative purposes.

4th century: Regular massages are administered to gladiators to ease muscle fatigue and pain. Julius Caesar is 'pinched' all over as a daily treatment for neuralgia.

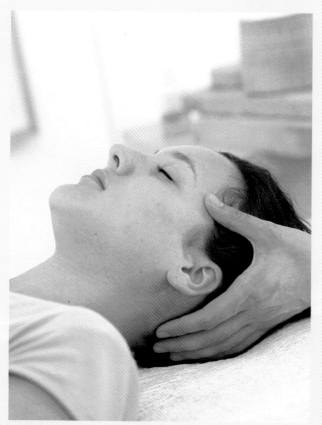

1st century AD: The Roman physician Tiberius declares that massage cures paralysis (more writings on this subject are published in the 17th and 19th centuries).

10th century: Avicenna, the canon of Arab philosopher and physician Ali Abu Ibn Szinna, tells of the health-promoting properties of massage combined with hydrotherapy, stating that it helps to disperse muscle by-products not expelled by exercise.

16th century: After suppression in the Middle Ages, massage makes a strong comeback. Many prominent physicians incorporate it into their approach, including the eminent Amrose Pare, medical advisor to four French kings.

18th century: The medical profession regains its prestige and massage takes a great leap forward worldwide, leading to abundant documentation on the subject. Captain Cook is adamant that massage received while visiting the Pacific Islands cured his sciatica.

19th century: The best-known development in massage takes place early this century. Per Henrik Ling, a Swedish gymnast, combines his knowledge of philosophy and gymnastics with massage techniques acquired during his travels to China. This combination of five basic strokes becomes known as the 'Swedish Movements' and is practised in much the same way today.

The use of the discipline spreads very quickly, with the first college offering massage on the curriculum established in 1813 and the first book in English on the Swedish Movements, written by Dr Mathias Roth, published in 1850.

20th century: The Military Massage Service is set up in 1914 and revived again in 1939 to help treat the war wounded.

The biggest turn round for massage comes in the 1960s and 1970s, with advocates considering it to be a powerful means by which to promote personal growth. This idea emanates from the Esalen Centre in California, where massage is used intuitively and in a truly holistic way, connecting mind, body and spirit and bringing us back full circle to how it all began over three thousand years ago.

So where do we stand now, in the 21st century? Massage has become a mainstream complementary therapy and also a part of integrated medicine as we know it. It is used throughout society on many levels and has a very important role to play in maintaining a healthy everyday life.

Preparation

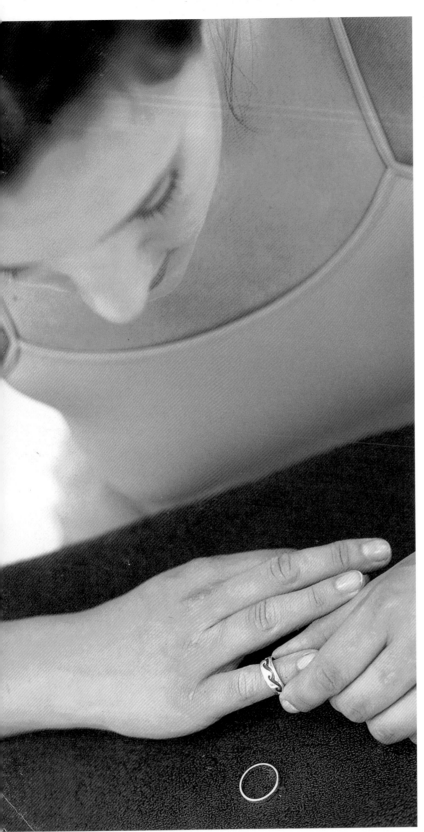

Massage is easy to learn: be guided by your instincts and you will be able to sense where to touch, how to touch and for how long. There are just a few basic guidelines to follow to ensure a comfortable and beneficial treatment. During massage there is an interaction of touch and response, which means that the giver has to prepare to give while the receiver must allow them to do so. Only then can this two-way flow be effective.

The Giver

You must choose to give your time to someone. If your mind is elsewhere and you would rather be watching television, your partner will sense this and the massage will not be pleasurable. Care, sensitivity and respect are very important requirements, so state of mind should be freed up to give your partner your full attention.

With this in mind, it is not a good idea to try to give a massage if you are feeling stressed or tense or if you are not in full health, as your energy level will be depleted. Both before and during the treatment, be aware of your breathing but do not try to change it.

Make sure you are wearing comfortable footwear and clothes. Choose something with short sleeves or roll them up out of the way. Try to remember to take off any noisy jewellry, which can be very distracting, and to remove your watch and any rings.

You cannot massage with long nails, and rough skin will feel very abrasive to the receiver, so get out the nail clippers and hand cream. Tie back any long hair that may get in the way. Remember that you will be working very close to your partner, so if you have recently indulged in food and drink that might have unpleasant after-effects on your breath be kind to your partner and use a mouthwash or breath freshener.

The Receiver

Believe it or not, it is often much more difficult to receive than to give: the ability to trust and let go sometimes also has to be learned. Be receptive to the touch, allow the giver to move your limbs for you when required, and let them know if anything is uncomfortable or when a stroke is particularly effective.

Sometimes massage can release pent-up emotions. If this happens, there is nothing wrong – do not fight the feeling or become embarrassed, but simply let them go.

Before the massage begins, remember to take off all your jewellry, including earrings, and if you are wearing contact lenses you may prefer to remove them for comfort and safety.

The main issue is what to wear. With close friends and family, you may be happy to undress to underpants; otherwise, only the areas of your body that are being worked on need be exposed at any one time. The ideal is to work free of clothing restrictions, but the massage environment is not always appropriate for this.

As with the giver, do not forget that fresh breath is a must, so use a mouthwash before your massage.

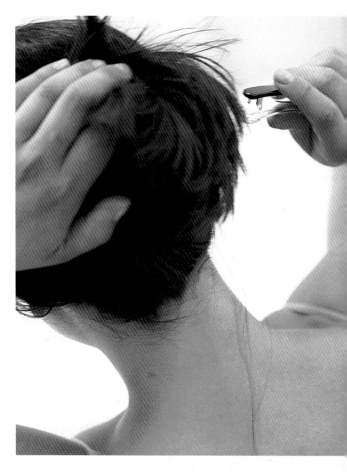

WHEN NOT TO MASSAGE

In general, massage is safe. Trained therapists are able to treat everyone from premature babies to the terminally ill, but there are nevertheless certain guidelines for you to observe. These include:

- Anyone weak or clinically exhausted – for example, suffering or recovering from a viral infection.
- Anyone who has a high temperature or is suffering from a contagious disease.
- Infectious skin complaints, such as scabies, herpes and warts.
- Serious medical conditions such as cancer, heart disorders or thrombosis.
- The site of a recent fracture, strain or sprain. In these cases, work one joint above.
- Where there are skin surface problems, such as scar tissue, bruising, tender or inflamed areas and varicose veins, do not work on them directly. You

can, however, work with care above the site and, of course, on other unaffected parts of the body.

- Do not massage during the first trimester of pregnancy and thereafter avoid very deep pressure, particularly on the lower back and inside leg from ankle to groin.
- After surgery, wait for 12 months following major operations and six months following minor procedures. Scar tissue should then be fully healed, but if in doubt seek medical practitioner approval.

It is also not advisable to receive massage if you have recently eaten a heavy meal or have been drinking quantities of alcohol, as this will make the experience very uncomfortable and may produce unpleasant after-effects. The general rule is to trust your own judgement and common sense and, if in any doubt, check with a doctor.

Oils, Lotions and Potions

Most massage treatments require the use of a lubricant to allow your hands to work smoothly and evenly over the skin without breaking the rhythm. This usually takes the form of oil, although lotions, creams and sometimes talcum powder can be used if you prefer.

How much lubricant you use will depend on the size of your partner, how hairy they are, and the dryness of their skin, but in general approximately 50ml (2½fl oz) is needed for a whole body. It may take a few tries to get it right: most people tend to use too much at first, which means you will not be able to make good contact. Your aim is to use just a thin film, which will be absorbed into the skin after the treatment.

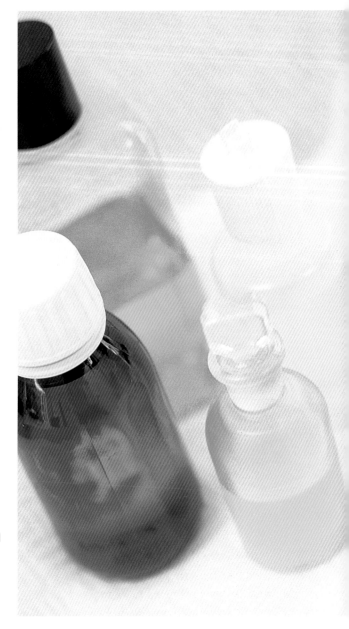

Household Oils

You can use oils that you keep at home in the kitchen cupboard – sunflower, grapeseed and vegetable oils all make excellent carrier or 'base' oils, as they are known professionally. If you want to pamper your partner, almond oil is a little costly but a real treat, particularly when used on the face. There is no need to worry about nut allergies because you are only applying oil externally and the penetration is superficial. However, some baby oils that include lanolin may cause an adverse skin reaction and tend to be absorbed less easily.

Essential oils

You may be tempted to rush out and buy aromatherapy or essential oils to add a further dimension to your massage. However, there are some cautions. These oils are very concentrated and powerful; many have contraindications, and unless you are a trained aromatherapist you should stick to the 'safe' oils, such as lavender and chamomile.

Never apply essential oils neat to the skin, but always mix with a carrier oil in the ratio of 1 drop essential oil to 2ml (scant ½ teaspoon) carrier oil. For example, 10ml (2 teaspoons) sunflower oil would allow you to use a maximum of 5 drops of essential oil. Mix only enough for the treatment, as oils exposed to the atmosphere oxidize and become rancid.

Store aromatherapy oils in dark bottles so as not to destroy their properties. Always read the instruction leaflets carefully, and if in doubt consult a trained aromatherapist or use plain oil.

There are now so many pre-blended oils available, covering all types of occasions and moods, that purchasing one of these is often the safest and most economical way of enhancing your massage treatment.

Lotions, Creams and Powders

Massage lotions and creams are also available, and these are pleasant to use on particularly dry skin or areas such as the feet. You may already have a plain emollient at home that can be used, but note that it is not advisable to massage with a cosmetic body lotion which may be too highly perfumed for the task. Talcum powder is another medium sometimes used by professionals – for reflexology in particular – and is perfect when applying strokes that do not require much glide.

Preparation

It is always best to prepare oils beforehand so that you do not interrupt the mood you are trying to create for the massage. The easiest and least messy method of dispensing oil is to keep it in a small plastic bottle with a flip top, which will reduce the likelihood of spillage. Alternatively, pour some oil into a small bowl into which you can dip your fingers easily. Most lotions, creams and powders are ready-packaged in suitable containers.

Another consideration for your partner is to warm the oil and your hands before making contact. If possible, place the oil container in hot water or close to a heater for a few minutes before starting the massage.

Applying Oil

1

There are various ways of applying oil. The most obvious is to pour about 2.5ml (½ teaspoon) of oil into the palm of one hand and then rub both palms together to spread the oil evenly. Do not be tempted to wring your hands as you might when washing or applying hand cream, because you want to oil the flat of your hands only. Make sure you apply the oil with your hands slightly away from your partner's body and then gently bring them down, ready to begin with a long application stroke.

2

The least intrusive way of applying more oil is to leave one hand on your partner's body, slowly pour the oil over the back of the hand and then glide the flat of your other hand across, spreading the oil on the body. A similar method is to turn your contact hand upwards and cup it, then pour oil into the palm – this has the added benefit of re-oiling both hands when you glide the other hand over.

Application and Contact

The confidence with which you make contact with your partner's skin and apply oil during massage is very important. The aim is for that first touch to feel relaxed and reassuring, transmitting the message that this is the start of the treatment and enabling your partner to get used to your touch. Most professional training teaches that you should not break contact with your partner during a massage, so one hand is placed on them throughout. When you work at home, this may prove difficult at first, especially if you are massaging on the floor. Simply make sure that if you need to break and re-establish contact you carry it out in a smooth, gentle manner, maintaining the flow of the massage and not leaving your partner wondering whether the treatment has finished. A good massage should have a definite beginning and end so that it feels complete – do not leave your partner with a sense that something was missing.

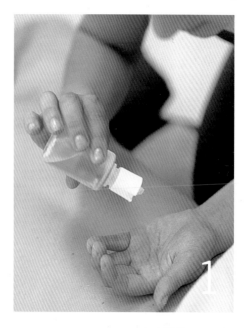

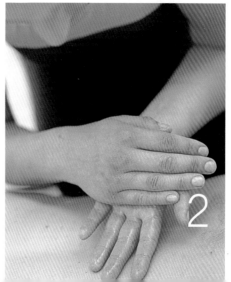

Creating a Relaxed Environment

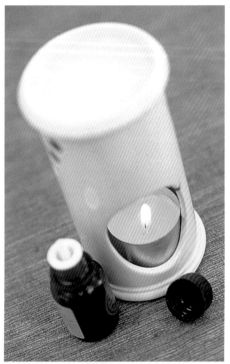

In later chapters you will see massage being performed in a range of environments, using techniques that are suitable with and without clothing, and working on floor, chair and table. Whichever of these you choose, preparing the surroundings is an important element in creating the atmosphere of comfort and relaxation that is central to any touch therapy. It does not matter what your home is like – a few simple touches can quickly transform almost any room into a place of calm and tranquillity.

Warmth

The most important consideration is heating. Body temperature drops while receiving massage, and muscles will not relax in a chilly atmosphere, so the room needs to be warm before the treatment begins. A little fresh air is good, but you should eliminate any draughts. Your partner will really appreciate if you use warm towels, which can be placed on a radiator or in an airing cupboard ready for use, and do not forget to take chill off the oil (see page 11).

Peace and Quiet

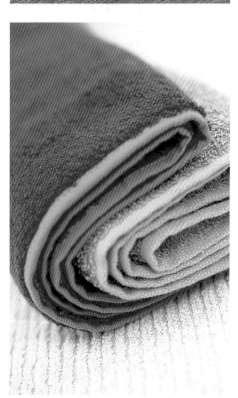

The next most important requirement is quiet. You will not relax into the massage if there is a television or radio playing in the background or if other members of the family are running in and out of the room. Choose a time when the children are occupied, put the telephone on answer service, switch off your mobile and give yourself and your partner this gift of time to relax and re-energize.

Having said this, some people like to have music playing, which helps both giver and receiver as they relax into the rhythm of the massage. There are many excellent CDs and cassettes available specifically for this purpose that you can try out. This idea is not new: centuries ago in Turkey massage often took place close to running water, as it was considered therapeutic to listen to its 'music'.

Lighting

Avoid direct lighting, as this can feel intrusive and you want your eyes to relax as much as the rest of your body. Depending on the time of day, subdued lights such as table lamps are ideal. Natural light can be good for the daytime, especially the morning, but you may wish to create a special feel in the evening by using candlelight or oil burners.

Fragrance

Make sure that the room has a pleasant aroma. This can be achieved with flowers, fragrant candles, essential oil burners or incense, but do make sure that your partner will not have an adverse reaction to whichever source of scent you choose. Select an aroma with which you are both happy or simply make sure you have a clean, fresh atmosphere by airing the room earlier in the day. Some people may even prefer quite a clinical environment. The main aim is to create a space in which both giver and receiver can relax.

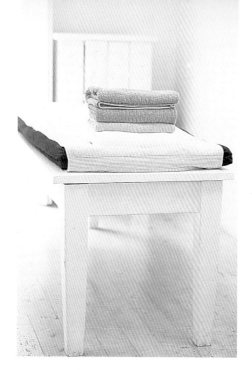

Equipment

Check that you have everything to hand before you start working so that you do not break your concentration. You will need:

- Your chosen oil
- Box of tissues or kitchen roll
- Two large bath towels or sheets
- Smaller hand towel
- Small cushions or a pillow
- Blanket or lightweight throw if the weather is cold
- Water to drink following the massage

Base of Support

If you are working on the floor, a futon – a Japanese mattress – is ideal, but a thick duvet or blankets make excellent substitutes. Make sure that whatever you use has enough space for your partner to be comfortable, plus extra to save your knees when moving around. Do not massage on a bed, as it does not provide the necessary support for the receiver and makes it impossible for you to move easily around their body.

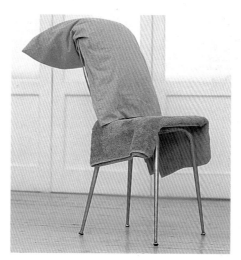

Cover the base with one large towel and use the other to cover your partner, only ever exposing the area of their body being worked upon. To retain the warmth of the muscles you may need to use a lightweight throw or blanket. A small towel can be used to cover a pillow if required, or it can be rolled up to offer support under the knees or ankles when needed. The general rule is to support the receiver's ankles when they are lying face down and their knees when they are face up.

If you have a sturdy table that can be adapted to a suitable height, width and length, you can place the padding on top and use this as a massage couch. To find the correct height, when standing straight, in the footwear you would be in when giving massage, drop your arms by your side and your knuckles should brush the top of the table. The table should be approximately 1.85m (6ft) long and about 65cm (26in) wide. You will find working on a table much less tiring than working on the floor, and it is easier to manoeuvre around without interrupting the flow of the massage.

If you find yourself massaging regularly, you might wish to invest in a professional couch. Most of these are lightweight, portable and easy to store away, folding up to the size of a large suitcase.

If you are working on a chair, choose one that is sturdy and stable and you will need to use a couple of pillows for comfort and support (see above for positioning of cushions).

The working positions and posture you should adopt for carrying out the various massage options are described on pages 22–7.

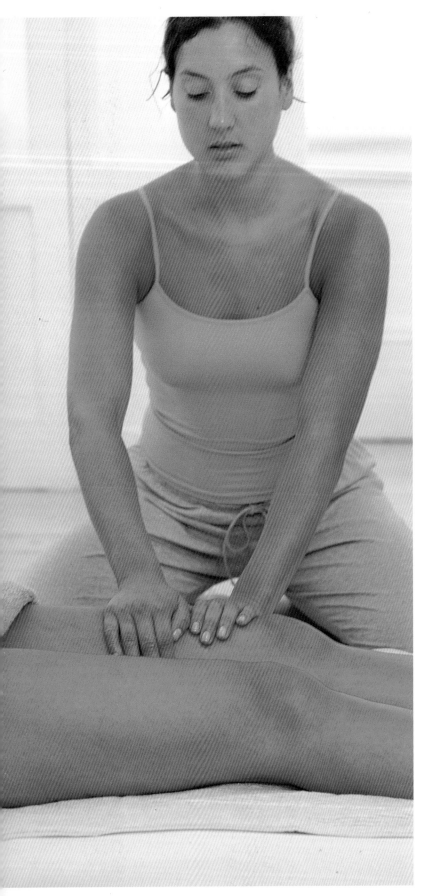

Anatomy

The more that you apply massage, the more you will be able to envisage what lies beneath your hands as they work. This in turn will stimulate your interest in learning about human anatomy and physiology. There are many good, user-friendly introductory books on the subject, but to start you on the path the following pages provide a simple overview, highlighting the main areas where most of the tensions and overuse occur, and relate to the massage routines outlined in later chapters.

The human skeleton comprises over 200 bones that have five main functions: support, protection, movement, storage and production. The muscles also work hard for us, performing many functions but primarily enabling us to move about, circulate blood, digest and breathe.

Massage can be effective at both the superficial and the deeper muscle levels: bodywork such as Rolfing claims to work on the muscle fascia itself. Massage can be used to relax or stimulate, and will also help to disperse knots of muscular spasm and toxins such as lactic acid.

Skeleton

The bones support the body and protect vital organs (as in the ribcage). They make movement possible with lever action at joints and the attachment of muscles. They also store nutrients and minerals, and produce red blood cells. Overall, bones are a very industrious body part and should be well cared for with good diet and exercise.

Joints are formed where two or more bones meet. They come in a variety of structures, from immobile links such as those in the skull to free-moving ones like those of the knee and elbow. There is also the ball-and-socket type, as at the shoulder and hip. The movement of free-moving joints is helped along by a lubricant called synovial fluid, which is secreted from a membrane lining a capsule that encases the ends of the bones, rather like oiling a hydraulic piston. Massage stimulates the production of this fluid, which is why sedentary and elderly people find regular treatments really help to sustain their mobility.

FRONT VIEW   **BACK VIEW**

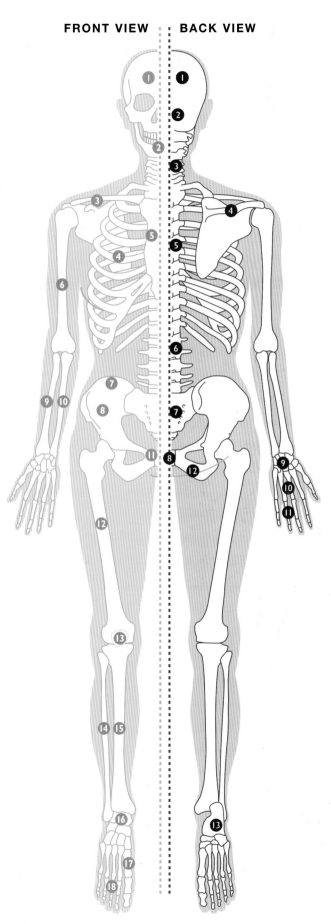

FRONT VIEW
1. cranium
2. mandible
3. clavicle
4. ribs
5. sternum
6. humerus
7. iliac crest
8. ilium
9. radius
10. ulna
11. pubic bone
12. femur
13. patella
14. fibula
15. tibia
16. tarsals
17. metatarsals
18. phalanges

BACK VIEW
1. parietal bone
2. occipital bone
3. cervical vertabrae
4. scapula
5. thoracis vertabrae
6. lumbar vertabrae
7. sacrum
8. coccyx
9. carpals
10. metacarpals
11. phalanges
12. ischial tuberosity
13. calcaneum

FRONT VIEW　　**BACK VIEW**

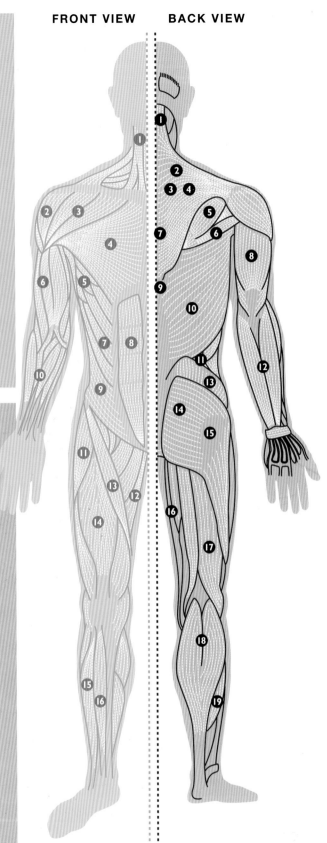

Muscles

There are two main muscle types: those that move automatically, such as the heart, which are called 'involuntary', and those you can move voluntarily with a message from the brain.

The muscles are arranged in layers, symmetrically on each side of the body. Each end is attached to a bone on either side of a joint – these are known as the 'origin' and the 'insertion' of the muscle. Most muscles move in pairs in opposite directions.

Muscles are made up of bundles of fibres or cells, fuelled by blood, lymph and nerves, and encased in fascia (connective tissue): imagine a telephone cable that has an outer casing and a multitude of smaller wires inside, and you will be picturing a muscle. The encased fibres slide between one another when instructed, causing the whole muscle to swell and shorten, which in turn causes the attached bones to move closer together – this process creates body movement. You may have heard the terms 'flexors' and 'extensors' – these are the muscles that, respectively, bend joints and straighten them.

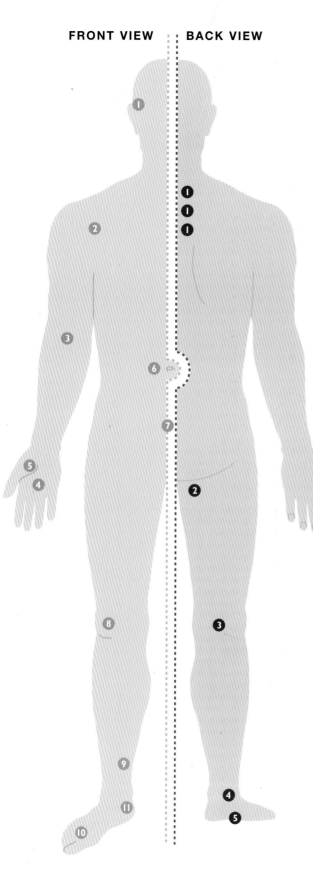

FRONT VIEW | BACK VIEW

Pressure Points

Pressure points are often used when massaging through the clothes. Work on these forms the basis of shiatsu (meaning 'finger pressure'), but can equally be incorporated into regular massage as a release mechanism for muscle tension. Working on these points stimulates the nervous system and gives out the signal to relax – rather like acupuncture without the use of needles. Pressure is applied with your thumb pad, although you can also use your elbow when working on the back area.

FRONT VIEW

❶ Side of head and hollows on outside edges of eye sockets *relieves migraine pain*

❷ Hollow at outer end of collarbone *stimulates lung function*

❸ Outside of end of elbow crease *relieves arm and shoulder pain and tonifies large intestine*

❹ Centre of palm *calms emotions and the mind*

❺ Web between thumb and index finger *eliminates colds, toothache and headache*

❻ About 7cm (3in) to either side of navel *relaxes stomach tension and aids digestion*

❼ Below navel, deep pressure with four flat fingers *stimulates whole body*

❽ Top of shinbone, in curve towards knee, *encourages well-being and energizes*

❾ Above inner ankle bone, four fingers up, *relieves menstrual pains*

❿ Between big toe and second toe, 3–5cm (1¼–2in) above join, *stabilizes liver function*

⓫ Inside heel at centre *stimulates kidneys*

BACK VIEW

❶ Either side of spine *brings equilibrium to body functions*

❷ Side of buttocks *relieves menstrual problems and relaxes pelvis*

❸ Back of knee (well supported) *relieves sciatica*

❹ Either side of Achilles tendon *stimulates water flow and relieves lower back*

❺ Under ball of foot *calms and relaxes generally*

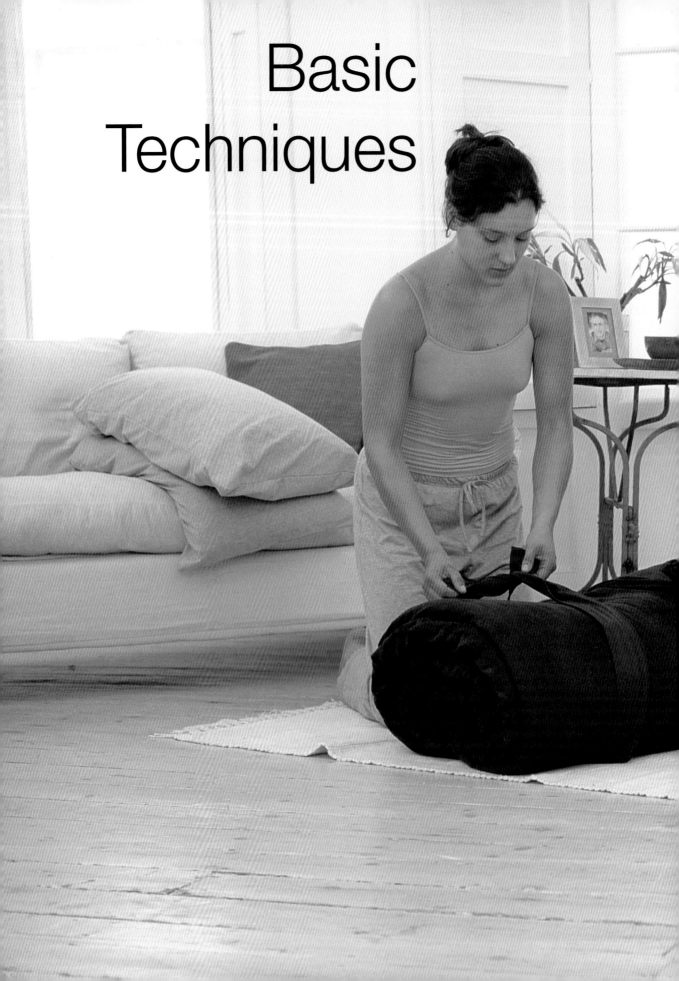

Basic Techniques

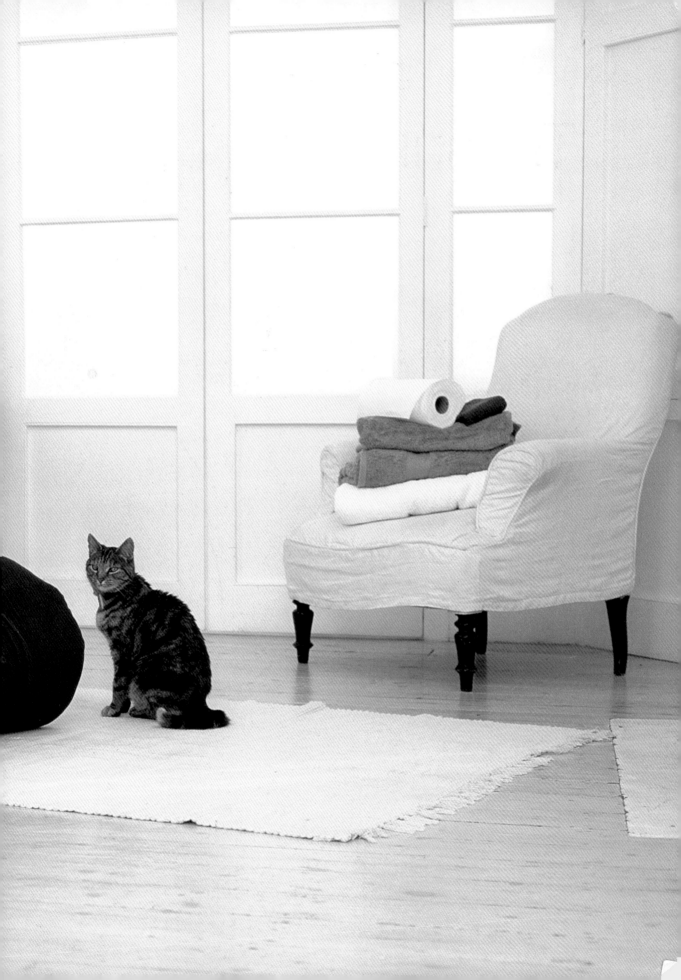

Giving Massage

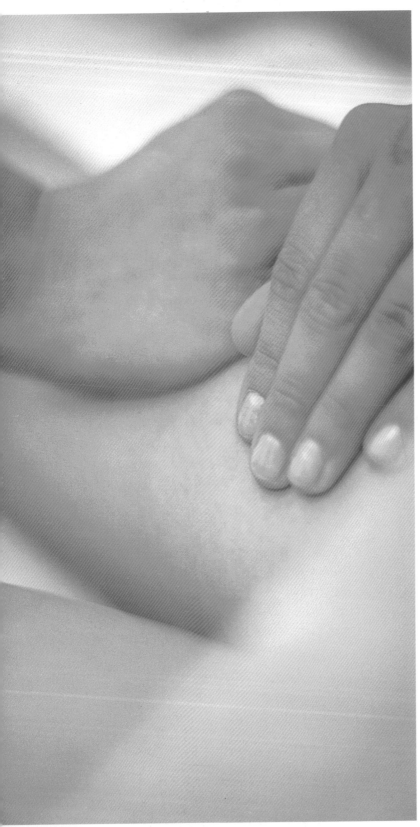

The techniques covered in this book are the 'mother' strokes of massage that are practised in the western hemisphere. Known as Swedish Massage, they consist of effleurage (gliding), petrissage (squeezing), tapotement (percussion), friction and stretching. These movements can be applied at different speeds and levels of pressure. However, the most important keys to a good massage are the rhythm and flow, so try to develop this sense and eventually you will not have to think about every stroke you are applying – they will come naturally. As the giver, try to think of the treatment as a dance.

In order for your partner to feel the full therapeutic benefits of a massage, the various strokes need to be applied in a specific order. Whatever length of treatment you are giving, you will always open by 'making contact', which sets the tone for the massage, followed by effleurage, which has several functions: to warm up the area for deeper work, to spread the oil or cream being used and to establish trust and confidence. You can then move on to the deeper work, using petrissage, percussion and friction once the muscles are relaxed and warm. If this preparation is omitted, strokes such as friction are not pleasant to receive. Finally, you will finish the massage with some stretching, more effleurage to calm the area and a 'holding' or 'grounding' technique which will also indicate to the receiver that the treatment is complete.

In general, massage strokes are applied working towards the heart, as in the venous flow. For example, if you are working on the

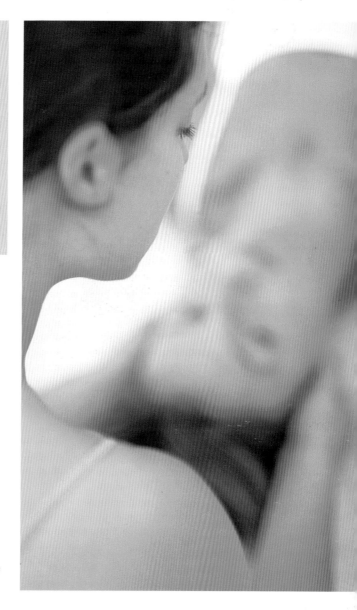

MASSAGE AREAS

A whole body massage is usually broken down into seven distinct areas.

Back
- torso
- legs and feet

Front
- face and scalp
- neck and shoulders
- arms and hands
- torso
- legs and feet

legs you will apply firmer pressure on the upward stroke and lighter pressure on the return stroke.

With your partner lying face down, your contact stroke is to place the flat of your hand confidently, and with good pressure, on the sacrum, then, using the strokes described later in this chapter, work over the whole of the back area, including the top of the buttocks and the lower back, the shoulderblades and the upper back, and, lastly, the sides of the torso. Make sure that you are careful not apply pressure directly to the spine, instead, work on either side of it.

After the back, move to the legs, working up from the ankle (reducing the pressure over the back of the knee joint) to the top and return, to finish on the foot.

Turn your partner over and begin with the shoulders, working on the back and front simultaneously. Move from the neck up to the scalp, then you are ready for the face routine. Next, massage each arm separately, working up the limb and returning, to finish with the wrist and hand. Next move on to the ribcage, the sides of the torso and the abdomen. Finish with the legs, once again working up from the ankle (avoiding pressure on the knee) to the top and returning, to finish on the foot.

Just as you start with 'contact', you need to end with 'connecting' or 'grounding' holds. You can either rest your hands on each foot with your thumbs placed on the instep area and apply medium pressure, or you can place your hands on two separate parts of the body – for example, the forehead and abdomen or the abdomen and feet.

A whole body massage should take 1–1½ hours, but as you become more proficient you may wish to concentrate on areas of tension or even give short treatments for remedial purposes. All these aspects are covered in this book.

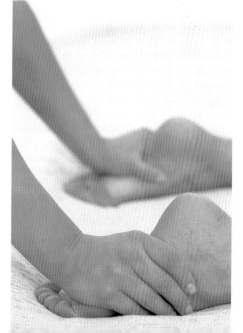

Posture and Position

Whether you are working with the receiver on a chair, the floor or a table, your own posture and position play an important part in the treatment by ensuring good control of rhythm, flow and pressure, and by keeping the physical effort required to a minimum so that the massage is pleasurable for both parties. A relaxed massage is as therapeutic to give as to receive, due to the exchange of energies involved. As the giver, your posture and position also need to be correct in order to avoid mechanical stress on your own body. This is taken very seriously by professional massage therapists, as their careers would be severely curtailed if they did not look after their own backs, arms and wrists.

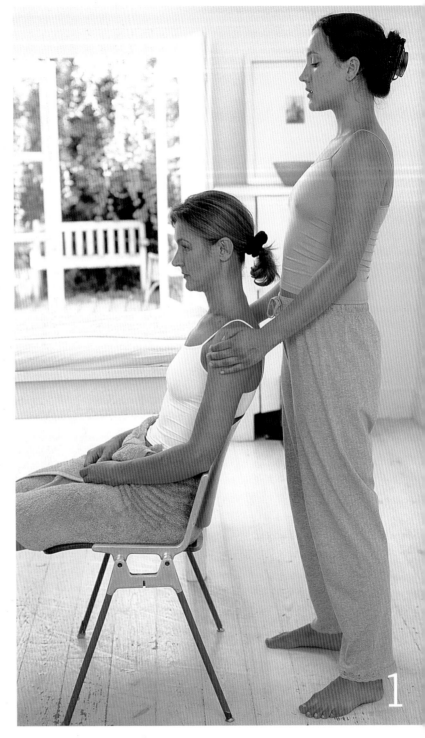

1

Chair

Some massage techniques can be carried out with the receiver sitting on a chair or stool. This is particularly useful when the floor is not comfortable for them, such as during pregnancy or for the elderly, and it is also

1

In the 'upright' posture, stand with your back straight, feet slightly apart and body weight balanced equally on both legs. The pressure required for the massage stroke is then directed through your arms, not your wrists, to the point of contact.

suitable for massaging in an office environment. There is no need for the receiver to undress, as most strokes can be applied through clothing or by rolling back the clothes (see page 9).

There are several positions the receiver can adopt for chair work:

- The receiver sits astride an upright chair, leaning into the back against pillows for padding and comfort, and resting their forearms and head on the top of the chair back (see page 13).

- The receiver sits naturally on the chair and leans forward onto a table or desk with a cushion for support (see page 100).

- The receiver sits upright in the chair when massage is being applied to the head, neck and shoulder areas from behind (see left and right) or to the arms, legs and feet from in front.

In all these instances, check that the receiver is well supported, that they have adjusted their position for comfort and that their back muscles are relaxed. Most importantly, always make sure that the chair is sturdy and safe.

As the giver, your stances are important to avoid any strain on your back. When you are working from the front, you can choose between kneeling, sitting or standing – whichever is most comfortable. When you are working from behind, you can use a combination of the 'upright' posture and the 'warrior' position.

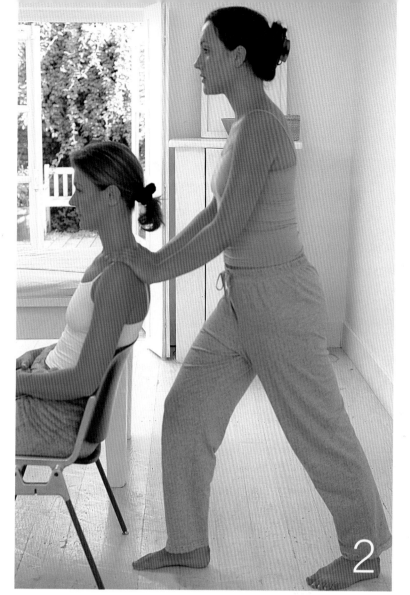

2

In the 'warrior' position – or 'to and fro' posture, as it is sometimes called – stand with your legs parallel but with one foot ahead of the other, toes facing forwards to provide a stable base. The further apart your feet are placed, the stronger the stroke. As you lean forward, applying pressure through your arms to the point of contact, you are also using your body weight behind the stroke by raising the heel of the back leg slightly, at the same time keeping the front leg relaxed. Your arms should be straight or flexed slightly at the elbow and your back more or less straight.

When you work with one hand only, your arm may be flexed at the elbow while the other arm is held straight with your hand placed suitably to maintain contact.

Floor

At home, you are most likely to be using the floor as your massage surface. A futon makes an ideal support for the receiver; otherwise, use a duvet, blankets or anything else suitable to provide some padding (see page 13).

Make sure you have enough space in which to move around easily without interrupting the flow of the treatment. If you are not positioned comfortably and are unable to relax, your partner will be able to sense this through the massage.

The main rules of posture for floor work are to:

- Relax your shoulders and upper back.
- Move from the hips and legs.
- As far as possible, keep your spine straight.
- Breathe!

Working on the floor requires more physical effort than working on a chair or table, so your positioning is important in order to conserve your energy.

To work at the top of the receiver's body, kneel 'astride' their head: as a guide, your knees should be parallel to your partner's ears. From here, you can drop your full weight into the point of contact by leaning directly over it, or directly backwards for stretching techniques.

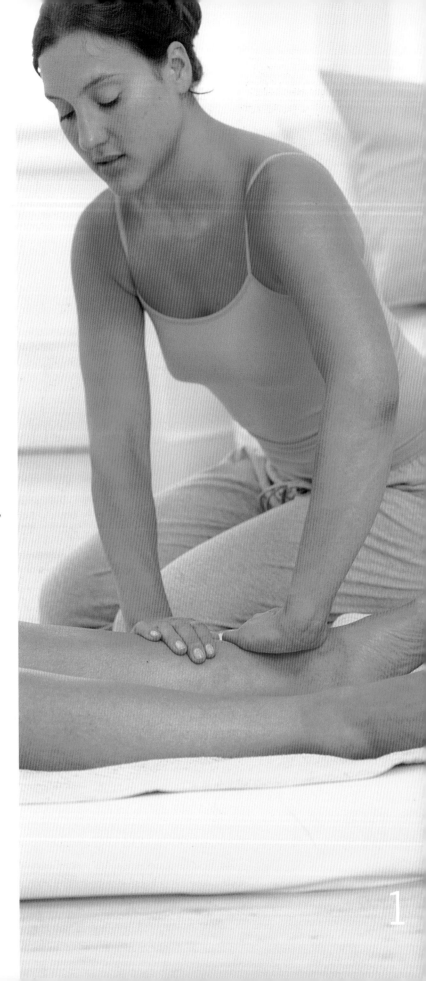

1

When working on areas such as the calves, thighs and sides of the torso, kneel side-on to your partner, with your knees apart and shoulders relaxed.

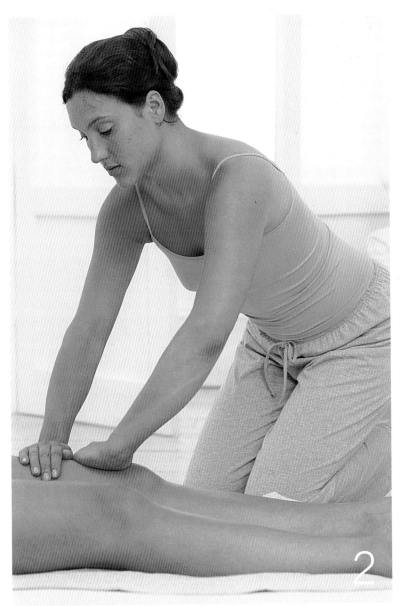

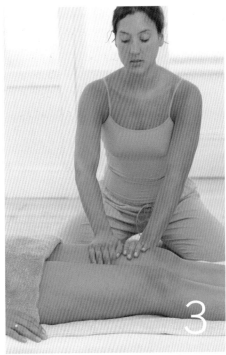

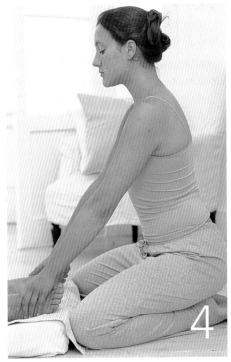

2

As you stretch forward, rise up slightly on your knees, moving from your hips and keeping your back and arms as straight as possible. Release on the return stroke.

3

For long, sweeping strokes up the legs or back, position yourself to one side of your partner, knees together and sitting back on your heels.

4

To work on the feet or for 'grounding' at the end of a treatment, adopt the same position side-on to your partner (see step 1), with your knees apart and shoulders relaxed.

Table

Using a table (see page 13 for dimensions) places less strain on your back and is not as physically demanding as working on the floor. You will also find it easier to move around. However, there is often a tendency to lean too far over your partner, so be aware of this and keep it in check.

The main rules for working on a table are:

- To stand square to the table.
- To bend from your knees and hips.
- Do not twist your body – always move from side to side or backwards and forwards using the postures shown.

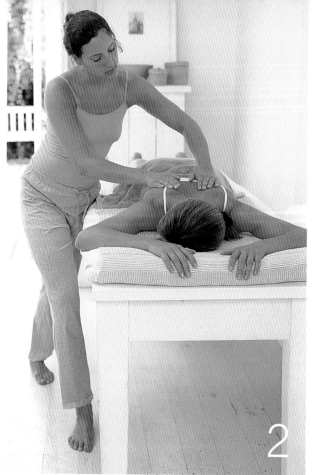

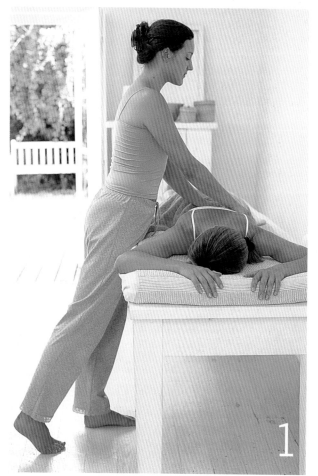

1

Use the warrior position (see page 23) when working at either end of the table or side on. This position allows you to determine the pressure of the stroke: the further apart your feet, the more body weight is transferred through your arms. The body movement in this position is backwards and forwards – as weight is shifted onto the front foot, the heel of the back foot rises slightly and the body weight transfers through the arms to the upward massage stroke. On the return stroke, the reverse happens.

2

The 'lunge' posture is used when you are working on either side of the table, enabling you to apply long strokes without having to bend your back. In this position you can lean against the table or position yourself slightly away from it, whichever is most comfortable. Keep both feet flat on the floor, then, as you move forwards, flex the front knee and keep the back leg straight. On the return movement you can choose to flex the back knee or keep it straight. Keep your arms straight when the stroke requires even pressure, but when working with one hand you can flex the elbow of the other arm slightly.

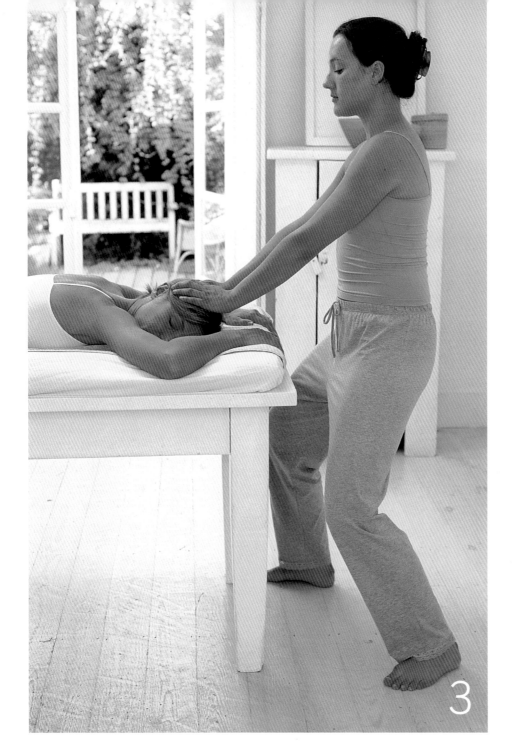

3

3

The 'monkey', or tai chi position, is used when a shift of pressure from one hand to the other is required and when strokes move from side to side rather than up and back. Standing slightly away from the table, place your body weight equally over both feet, with your knees slightly flexed and your back and arms straight. Shift your weight from one foot to the other to produce a side-to-side movement, which can be exaggerated or very slight depending on what is required. This position, with legs straight instead of flexed, is the upright position often used at the head or foot of the table.

Effleurage

A French word meaning 'stroking', effleurage is the simplest technique to perform and can be used everywhere on the body. It is a rhythmic movement, which is used especially to:

- Make and break contact.
- Enable your partner to relax under your touch.
- Enable you to sense areas of tension.
- Spread massage oil, lotion, cream or talcum powder.
- Connect different parts of the body.
- Warm the muscles in preparation for deeper work.

Effleurage also helps to improve blood and lymph flows and induces relaxation. In particular, it is the main stroke used to bring out the aromatherapeutic benefits of essential oils.

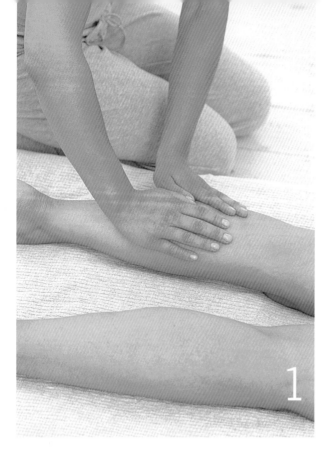

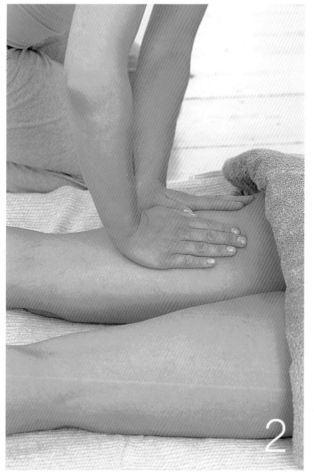

1 & 2 Flat-handed

Oil the flat of your hands and, with your fingers together and wrists relaxed, make contact with your partner and glide both hands simultaneously with pressure and momentum upwards to your natural reach, then separate and return along the sides of the limb or torso in a breaststroke-like movement. Repeat several times. Always remember to lift off pressure over joint areas, and when you work on the back place your hands on either side of the spine – do not work directly on it. Another way of administering this stroke on the back area is to make broad, circular movements, spiralling up to the shoulders and returning flat-handed down the sides. For extra pressure, one hand can be placed on top of the other to administer the stroke – this is known as 'double-handed' or 'reinforced' effleurage. Pressure can also be applied on the thumb only.

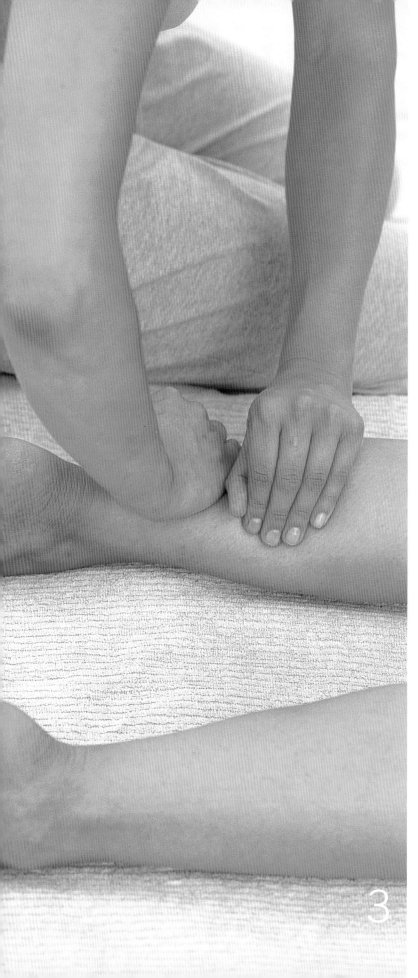

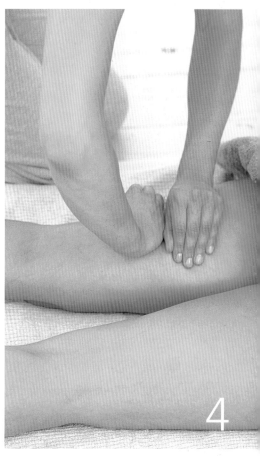

3 & 4 Cupped

This variation, in which the hands are cupped and horizontal, one above the other, is especially useful when you are working on the legs and arms. Oil your hands, then make contact with your partner and glide up the limb to your natural reach, turn and use the flat-handed stroke to return. Cupped effleurage is a very soothing stroke for the calf and arm muscles, which are often very sensitive areas. When working on the upper thigh, take the stroke further with the outside hand, turning the inside hand discreetly on your partner's inner thigh so as not to be intrusive.

Both flat-handed and cupped effleurage can be done in reverse, keeping the pressure on the upward stroke. This will work the muscle in a different way and feel quite different to the receiver.

Petrissage

Petrissage is the general name given to any stroke that presses, squeezes and rolls the muscles under the skin. It also includes kneading and wringing techniques. This is a medium-depth stroke that is used after effleurage, and it acts to:

- 'Milk' the muscles of waste products, literally squeezing the tension, toxins and tiredness out of the body.
- Prepare for deeper work, such as friction (see page 34).
- Break up specific knots of tension where appropriate.
- Stretch and loosen muscle fibres and fascia.
- Stimulate circulation to an area.

Petrissage also helps the blood and oxygen return, and to relax the muscles.

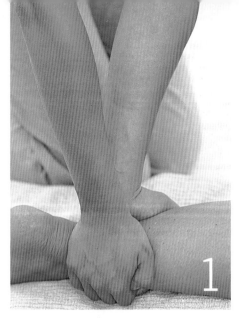

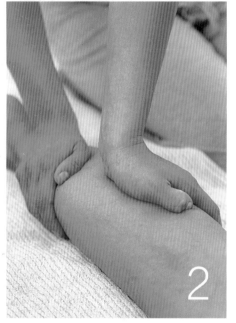

1

With your hands on top of the muscle and supporting the underside with your fingertips, squeeze the heel of your hands downwards, each hand mirroring the other, and then bring your fingers upwards so that you have a handful of flesh between the two. Slide the heel of your hands back and repeat in a continuous rhythm of squeezing and releasing, working upwards over the muscle.

2

Using the same procedure, you can work your hands alternately – one hand squeezing downwards and stretching upwards, followed by the other. On a larger area, such as the sides of the buttocks, this is particularly useful for working on one side at a time side-on.

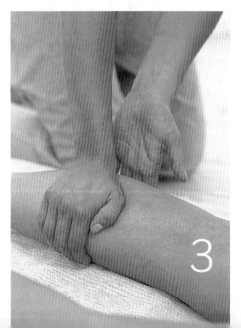

3

One-handed petrissage is most effective when strong pressure is required or when you are working on your partner's shoulders or along their back on either side of the spine. With one hand resting on the limb or torso, repeat the petrissage action with the other, sweeping over the muscle and adjusting the pressure according to your partner's tension.

1 Wringing

This is a stroke that literally 'wrings' out the tension and toxins stored in muscles. Using the whole of your hand with the thumb closed to the fingers, work alternately backwards and forwards in a continuous flow, lifting the skin towards you with one hand and pushing it away with the other. Wringing is mostly used on the calf and thigh, but if you are working on small muscles you can open your thumbs wide to get a firm grip as you wring.

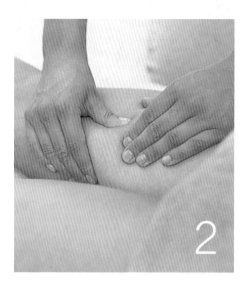

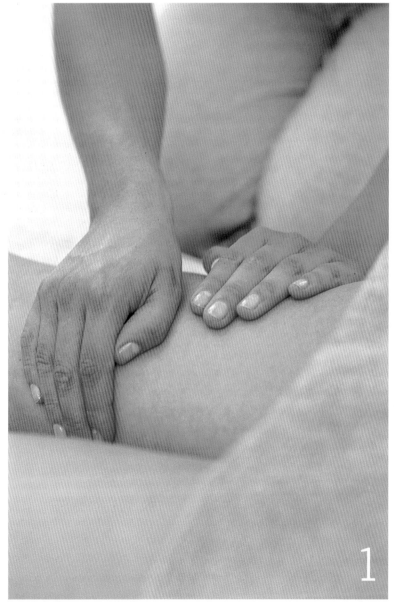

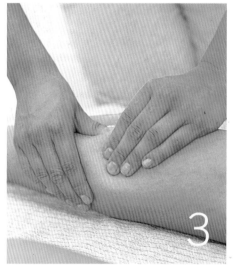

2 & 3 Kneading

Kneading, often mistaken as the only stroke of petrissage, requires medium pressure and should be applied only after the muscle has been relaxed, usually over large, fleshy areas. The slower and deeper the stroke, the more beneficial it is. Using the whole of your hand with the thumb spread, lean your hands firmly into the muscle and use them alternately, working them towards each other, squeezing and rolling the muscle in a side-to-side action – imagine you are kneading dough. Work your way up the muscle, keeping contact with both hands in a continuous, rhythmic motion.

Percussion

Percussion, named after the noise it makes, is known by professionals as tapotement, the French word for 'light tapping'. It consists of brisk strokes that are made by using both hands alternately in a rhythmic motion. As with the percussion section of an orchestra, the strokes build up slowly to a crescendo and then end abruptly. The technique is used to:

- Improve local circulation.
- Tone and stimulate soft tissue areas, such as the outer thighs and buttocks.
- Stimulate nerve endings.

No oils or creams are necessary to perform any percussive stroke.

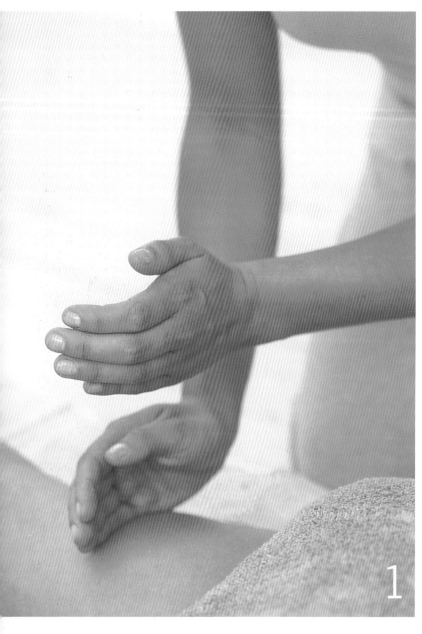

1 Hacking

Make sure your hands and wrists are relaxed by stroking and shaking them. In a chopping movement and with a flick of the wrists, bring your hands down alternately 4–5cm (1½–2in) apart onto your partner's body surface. Only the little finger should hit the tissue, with the other fingers cascading onto it, rising rapidly as the other hand descends. It may take a little practice to develop a smooth rhythm – try working in time to music with a good drum beat. Once you are proficient, you can vary the pace and strength of hacking according to your partner's requirements. A heavier hacking stroke can be applied with your fingers curled and closed together. Always keep your shoulders and elbows relaxed.

SAFETY FIRST

Take care when using percussive strokes, because they are not suitable for bony areas, the spine, head and neck, or the back of the knee. Nor should they be used where there is any inflammation, strain, paralysed muscle or varicose veins, or in the kidney area.

2 Pummelling

Lightweight pummelling – or pounding, as it is sometimes called – is performed (in the same way as other percussive strokes) with a flick of the wrist. For heavier work, the wrist is locked and the elbow bent, lowering the forearm and thereby providing more body weight behind the stoke. Make your hands into loose fists with your thumbs on top, then bring them down alternately, as in the hacking movement, with the fleshy (palmar) side bouncing firmly on the tissue and making a strong, rhythmic beating sound. This stroke is usually applied only to large, well-padded areas of muscle such as the buttocks and thighs.

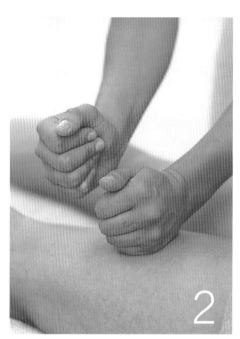

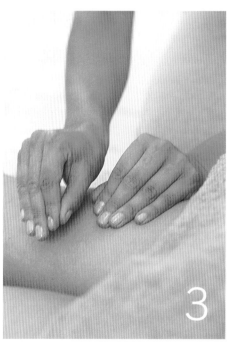

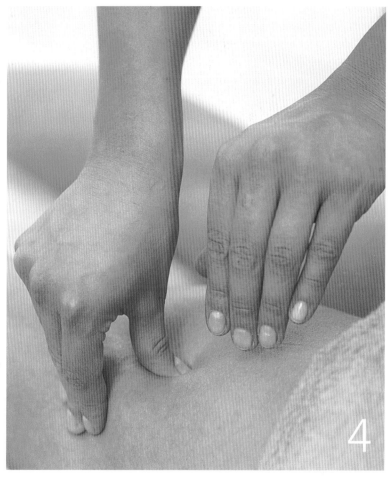

3 Cupping

Make a cup shape with your hands, keeping your fingers straight. Moving from your forearm, not your wrist, bring your hands down alternately onto your partner's body surface, trapping air against the skin and releasing it as you lift the working hand to 4–5cm (1½–2in) above the skin while dropping the other. This will make a hollow noise (similar to that of horses' hooves) as you work across the area.

4 Flicking

This technique is sometimes called plucking. With straight fingers, bring your thumbs and fingertips down onto your partner's body surface and, in a quick action, take up a small piece of flesh and then let it slip easily away with each stroke, turning your wrist very slightly as you release. Use your hands alternately in a steady, rhythmic motion.

Friction

A deep and focused stroke, friction is carried out following the warm-up strokes of effleurage and petrissage. The stroke uses mainly the fingertips, thumbs and heel of the hands, and is often done with only one hand at a time and with little or no gliding, so that oils and creams are rarely needed. Working in various directions, the movements reach deep down into the tissue where more tensions may be hidden. Friction is used to:

- Reduce oedema (water retention).
- Stretch and release knots of tension.
- Disperse calcifications around joint areas
  – as in gout for example.
- Stimulate the digestive tract and colon.
- Treat intense, intermittent pain from branches
  of the main nervous system.

SAFETY FIRST

Take care when using friction, and do not apply if the nerve is inflamed or on any area that reacts with a protective contraction. In particular, friction must be carried out gently and stopped immediately if nerve pain is exacerbated, as it will be counterproductive to overstep the mark.

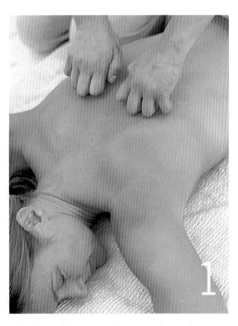

1 Straight Knuckling

Curl your hands into a loose fist and, with the knuckles flat on your partner's skin, glide up the leg or back using the middle section of your fingers. Do not rotate your fingers and always work towards the heart to aid blood and lymph flows. This stroke works deep into the muscle and tissue to release stubborn tensions and deposits.

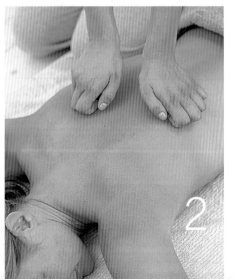

2 Circular Knuckling

As for straight knuckling, curl your hands into a loose fist, but instead of straight gliding, rotate the fingers at the same time to make a circular movement. This stroke is very pleasant to receive on the backs of the hands and the feet. Performed lightly to relax the chest and shoulder areas, you can also use it to work deep into the pectoral muscles or around the shoulder blade to release long-standing tensions.

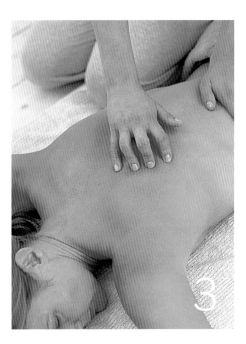

3 Circular Friction

For this stroke, work with one hand at a time, resting the other on your partner for reassurance. With your fingers slightly apart, apply even pressure through your fingertips by moving the tissues over the body's structure in a small, circular movement that starts gently and increases progressively. You can also work your fingertips backwards and forwards in a 'transverse' friction movement.

4 Thumb Rolling

Using the length of your thumbs and leaning into your partner's skin with your whole body weight, bring one thumb down behind the other, pushing away with short, deep strokes in a rhythmic motion. This stroke can be applied on small or large areas alike to smooth out knotty muscle fibres, and it is especially useful in reaching tension between the spine and shoulder blades.

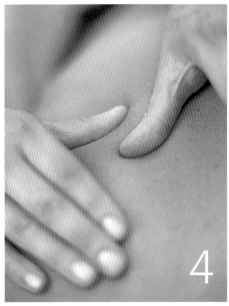

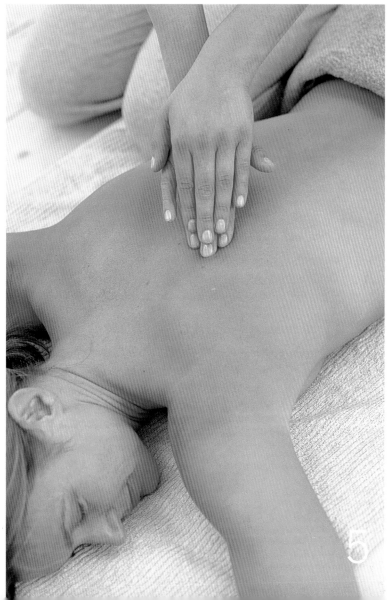

5 Circling

Place one hand on top of the other with your fingers straight but relaxed. Lean into the muscle with your fingertips and slowly make tiny circles, working around the joints and areas of tension. The aim is to move the underlying tissue rather than glide over the surface of the skin. On the back, work on the nerves and muscles that extend outwards from the spine. When circling the knee, use thumbs rather than fingertips.

Passive Stretching

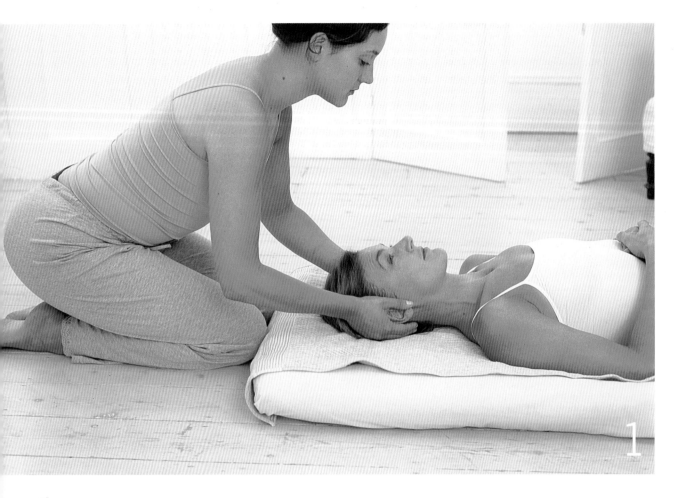

1

1 Head and neck

Position yourself at your partner's head and, with a hand on each side of the head, cup underneath the neck with the web of your hand and thumb around the ear. Make sure your partner is comfortable and then slowly pull back towards yourself, sliding your hands to the base of the skull. Relax and then repeat, making sure you do not pull from your shoulders and that your arms are relaxed. You can apply the same method to the legs by gripping the feet in a similar way.

During a massage it can be beneficial to include some passive stretching – which is rather like yoga without the effort! The technique involves extending the muscle to its natural resting length and holding this position for about 15 seconds before returning it to its shortest resting position, then repeating if necessary. Stretching goes right back to the roots of Western-style massage and it was employed by Per Ling in his original Swedish Massage technique. It is mostly restricted to the limbs and to a few conditions that are treated with massage. Make sure your partner is aware of what you are going to do, as this will help them to relax and work with you instead of resisting.

2 Ribcage

Slowly 'walk' your hands down your partner's arms until you reach the wrists, take hold firmly and lift the arms up slowly towards you. Breathe in, and on the out breath lean back slowly, taking your partner's arms with you. Make sure that the stretch is comfortable but effective. Hold this position for 15–20 seconds and release slowly. Repeat if required, increasing the stretch. This will expand the ribcage and stretch the respiratory muscles as well as the arm muscles.

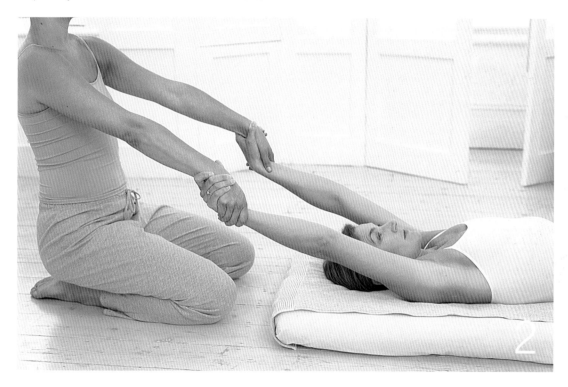

3 Arms

Working side-on to your partner, lift their arm with one hand and place it over your other arm, crooking it for support. Take hold of their wrist and smoothly lift the arm upwards, pulling it out towards you at the same time in a lift-and-pull movement. Lower and repeat, increasing the stretch each time. Repeat on the other side.

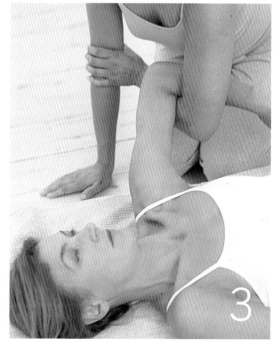

Completing the Massage

At the end of a massage treatment your partner will be feeling somewhat distant and relaxed, so it is very important to finish in a sensitive manner by bringing their awareness back slowly. However you begin your massage always finish with a grounding stroke to complete the routine and encourage your partner to stay still and rest for a few minutes before slowly getting up.

1 Feathering

This stroke is used when completing a massage sequence to soothe and calm, leaving your partner relaxed. Keeping your arms and hands relaxed, stroke your partner's skin lightly downwards, using one hand after the other and covering the maximum area without changing position. With each stroke lighten the contact until you are feathering slightly above the skin.

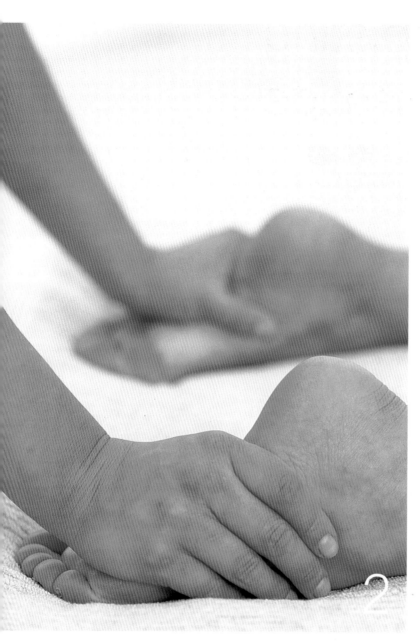

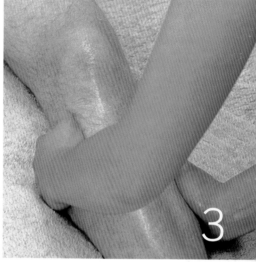

2 Grounding

At the end of a massage treatment the receiver may often feel quite distant, and it is important to bring their awareness back slowly. So, no matter how you begin your massage, always finish by holding the feet for at least 30 seconds, placing your thumb on the instep and the web and palm of your hand on the front or sole of the foot, employing a strong, even pressure. If you have been working on the upper body only, grounding will also help to 'reconnect' the receiver, completing the massage in a caring, holistic way and indicating to your partner that this is the end of the treatment.

3 Rocking

This light pressure stroke is used after working on a particular area of the body, or early in the massage to relax and loosen the limbs, encouraging your partner's body to let go and succumb to the treatment. When working on the arms, face up your partner's body and support the upper arm by cupping your hands on either side. Rock the arm back and forth between your hands, slowly moving down the arm and increasing the pace around the wrist area. Finish by stroking over the fingers. Repeat on the opposite arm.

To rock the legs, stand or kneel at your partner's feet, facing up their body, and place your hands on either side of the thigh. Rock the leg back and forth between your hands, moving slowly down the leg, and finish by stroking over the toes. Repeat on the opposite leg. If you are at the end of a massage treatment, end by grounding your partner.

Using Massage Aids

In recent years massage has become a mainstream therapy that most people have heard of, even if they have not already tried it for themselves. To meet demand, many stores and websites now stock a variety of massage tools, both manual and electric, to enhance your massage skills. Here is a small selection of favourites that are widely available, plus some interesting substitutes that you may already have lying around the house.

1 & 2

This is great for massaging arms and thighs and self-massaging the shoulders, although a simple pine cone will have a similar effect.

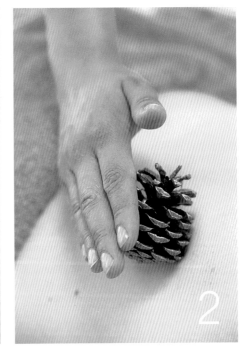

1

2

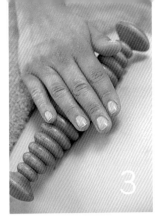
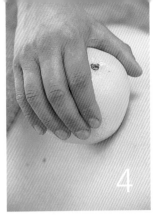
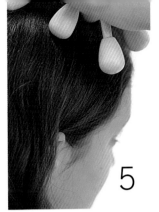
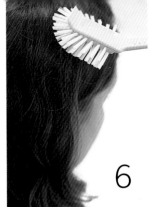

3 & 4

A wooden roller ball works wonders on the back and shoulder blades, but a grapefruit will feel just as good and the aroma has uplifting properties for you to inhale as you work.

5 & 6

These cute wooden ladybird massagers give a great scalp massage and are very invigorating – but so is your washing-up brush.

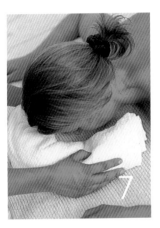

7

To make your partner more comfortable when they are lying on their front, roll up a hand towel and make it into a horseshoe shape to support their face. A massage therapist may use a face cradle made specially for this purpose. This fits onto the end of a massage table, allowing easier access to the neck and shoulder area.

8

When your partner is lying on their front their ankles will need support. Fold up a small towel and, taking the ankle securely, gently lift each foot so that you can position the towel. When lying on their back, they may also wish to have their knees supported to take the pressure off the lower back area. Again using the rolled-up towel, lift each knee and replace when you position the towel. If you start to massage regularly, you may wish to buy a purpose-made bolster or even make your own.

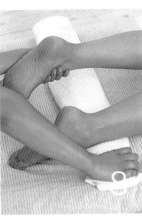
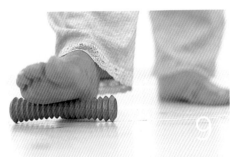
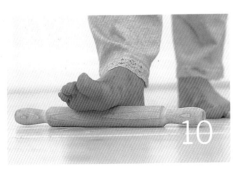

9 & 10

A wooden foot roller can be used on other areas of the body, or you can use a pastry rolling pin to do the job instead.

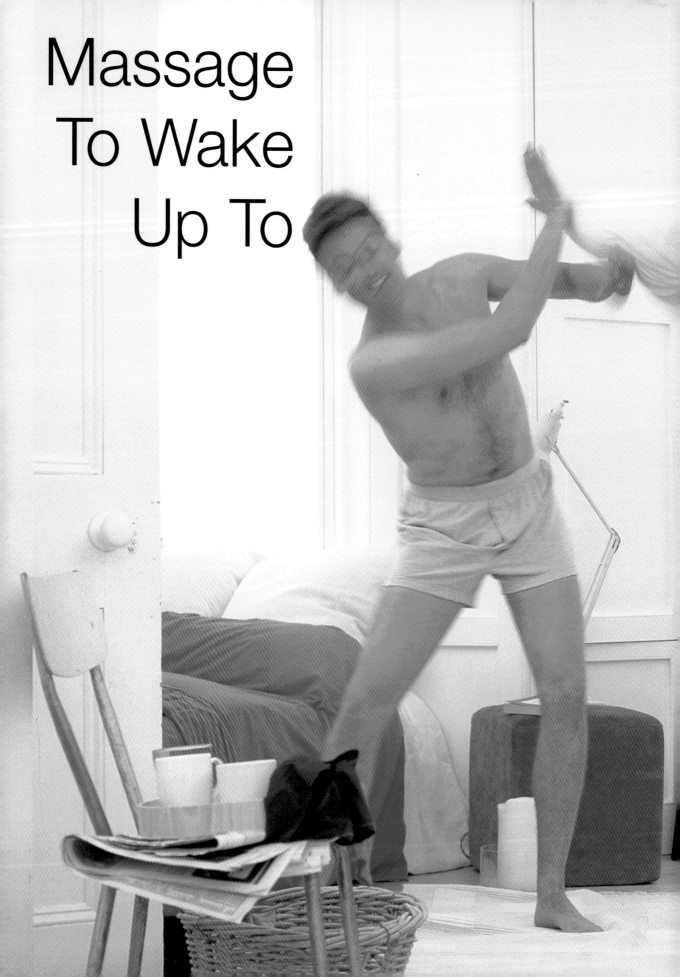

Massage
To Wake
Up To

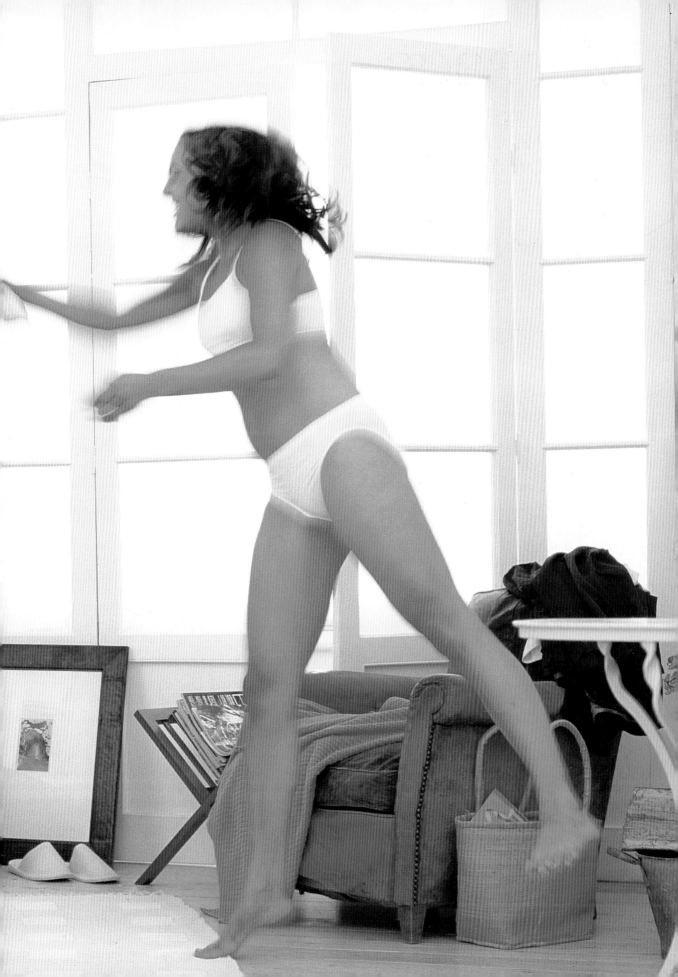

Percussion and Friction

Many people think that massage is just for relaxing and is therefore ideal before bedtime, but it can be used at all times of the day and be either stimulating or relaxing – rather like choosing between a shower and a bath. To get all your systems moving in the morning, strokes such as percussion and friction are used to stimulate the blood and the lymph flows, ready for the day's action.

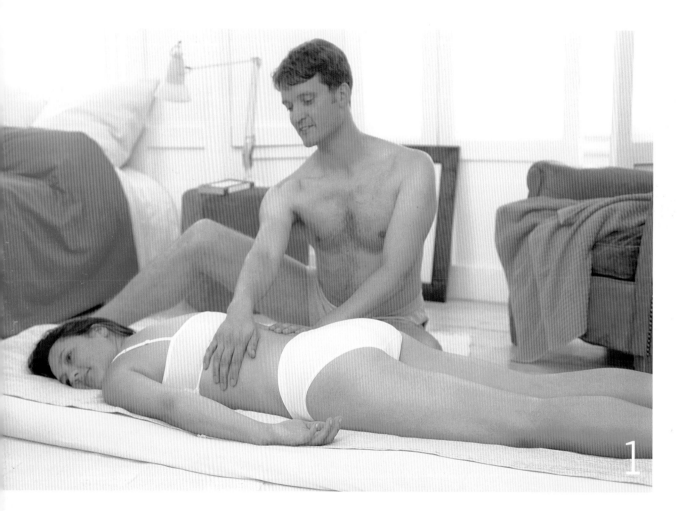

1

1

With your partner lying face down, position yourself side-on and with both hands apply the wringing stroke (see page 31) across the whole back. Place one hand on the side of the back nearer to you and the other on the far side, then push forwards with the heel of the nearside hand while pulling back with the fingers of the other, working in a continual criss-cross movement.

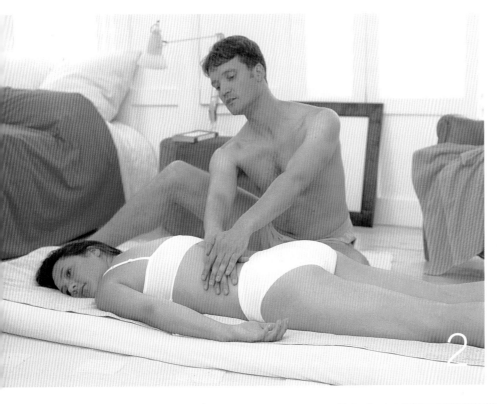

2

With one hand palm down on your partner's back, place your other hand on top and, using the effleurage stroke (see page 28), glide in large, circular movements over the whole of the back area.

3

Using the flicking movement (see page 33), work all over the shoulder blade area, avoiding the spine. This will stimulate the circulation and help to clear the lungs of any congestion.

SAFETY FIRST

Remember: always work on either side of the spine, never directly over it.

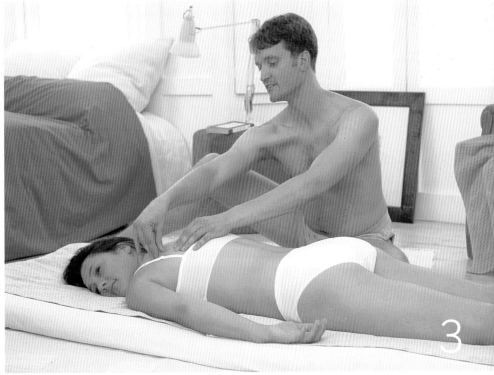

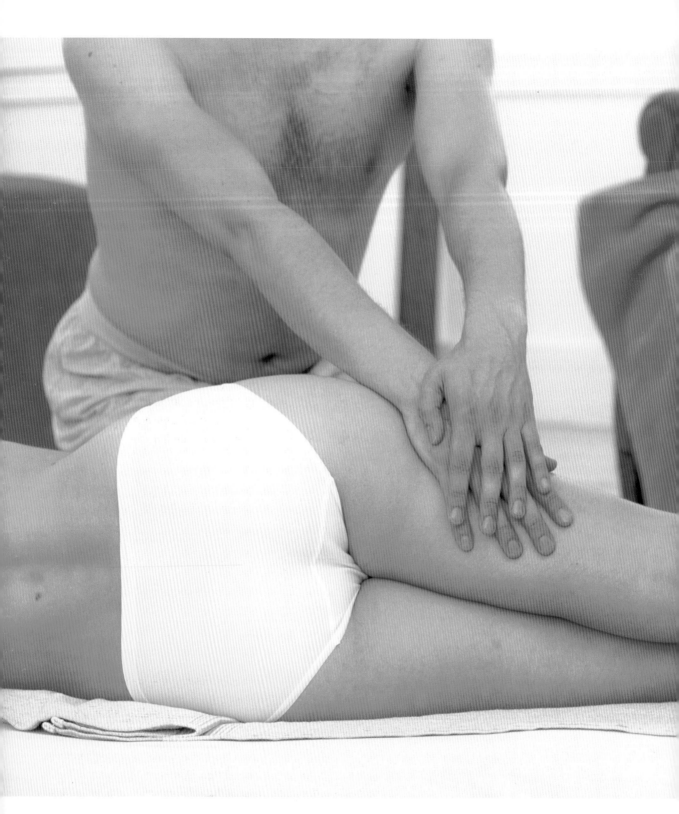

4

With your partner lying comfortably on their side, use the double-handed effleurage stroke in step 2 to massage over the whole of the back of the upper leg and thigh.

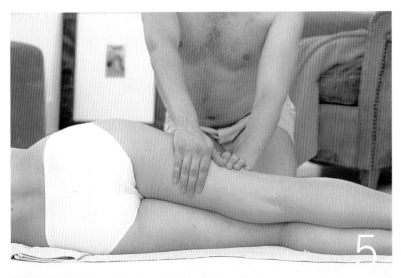

5

With your partner in the same position and making sure that the leg is supported, use the wringing stroke as in step 1 to work over the top of the leg between the knee and the hip.

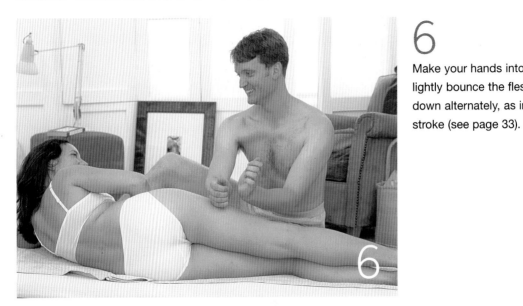

6

Make your hands into loose fists and lightly bounce the fleshy sides up and down alternately, as in the pummelling stroke (see page 33).

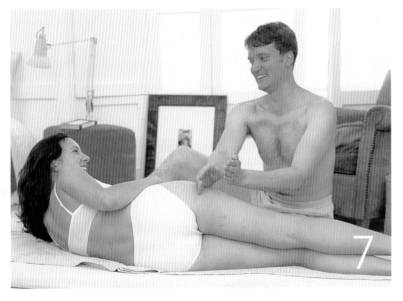

7

After completing the pummelling, shake your hands to relax them. In a movement similar to step 6 but with your hands open and relaxed, bring down the the edge of each hand alternately, slowly gathering momentum. Once you have established a good, sustainable rhythm, work on the muscle directly. This is the hacking stroke (see page 32).

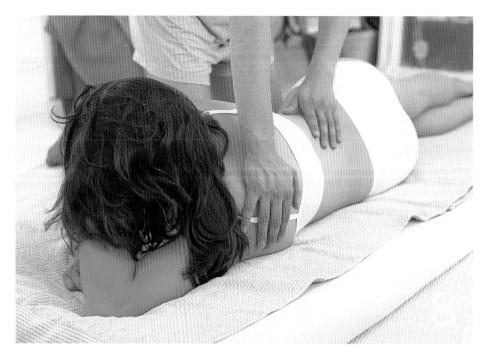

8

Place one hand on your partner's shoulder furthest away from you and the other on the nearer lower back. Push forward with the heel of the hand on the shoulder, at the same time pulling back with the fingers on the opposite hand, thereby facilitating a long stretch diagonally across the length of the torso. Exchange hands and sides, and repeat.

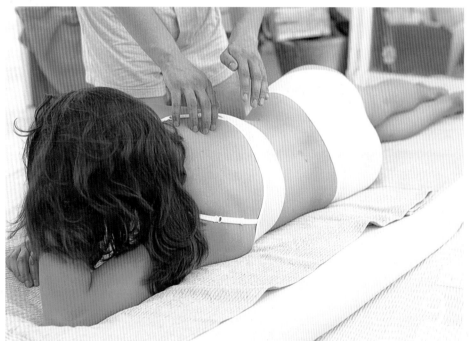

9

Using the tops of your fingers in rotation, tap your partner's skin in such a way that only one finger is touching at a time. Use both hands simultaneously and increase the speed but not the pressure. Using this tapping motion, work over the muscles between the shoulder blade and the spine to relieve any congestion in the lung area.

10

This is another variation on the hacking stroke (see page 32), called 'open-handed hacking'. The fingers are spread apart to give a lighter pressure and sensation. Using this stroke, work all over the back area, avoiding the spine, to stimulate blood circulation and to get everything moving for the day ahead.

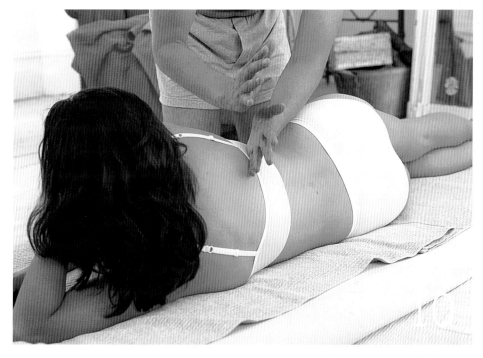

11

This dynamic use of the hacking stroke is taken from Indian Ayurvedic massage, in which it is applied to the head. Work lightly over the whole of your partner's scalp to stimulate blood flow. This technique is also extremely beneficial in encouraging hair growth and condition.

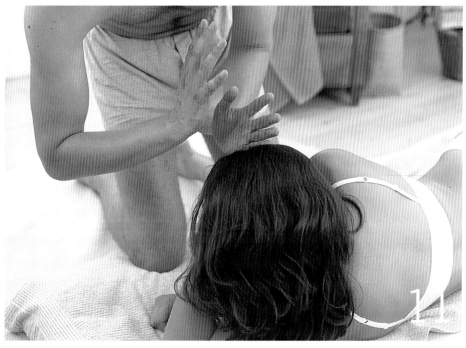

Pressing and Drainage

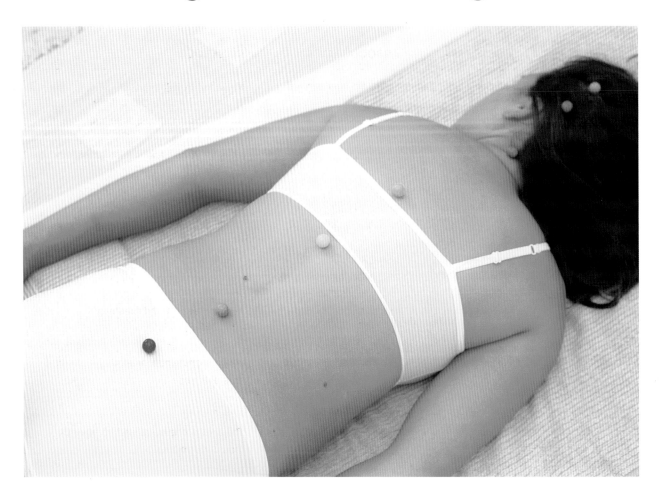

Eastern practitioners believe that the body contains seven main energy centres, or spinning wheels, called chakras, the Sanskrit word for wheel. These are positioned along the length of the spine and can be sensed from the back and front alike. Each chakra is connected to a particular part of the body and has its own colour association and emotional attributes. Balance between the seven chakras results in maximum health and vitality, and massage helps to restore this balance.

1

With the pads of your thumbs, press down on the root chakra at the base of the spine, hold for three to five seconds and release. Repeat twice.

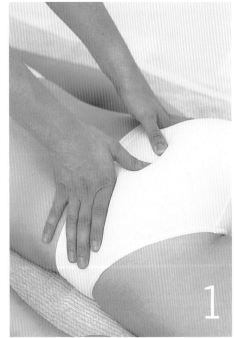

THE SEVEN CHAKRAS

Working upwards from the base of the spine, the seven chakras are:

CHAKRA	COLOUR	ASSOCIATION	CONTROLS
1 Root chakra	red	will to be and survival	legs, feet and gonads The root chakra is the base for all the others and so affects their balance.
2 Sacral chakra or hara	orange	vitality and sexuality	adrenal glands and digestive system
3 Solar plexus	yellow	personal power and raw emotion	pancreas
4 Heart	green	heart, circulation and lower lungs	love and compassion
5 Throat	blue	lungs, throat and respiratory system	self-expression and creativity, often linked
6 Brow or 'third eye'	indigo	intuition and intellect	nervous system, forehead, ears and nose
7 Crown	violet	superconsciousness and spirituality	pineal gland The crown chakra is said to have a thousand petals.

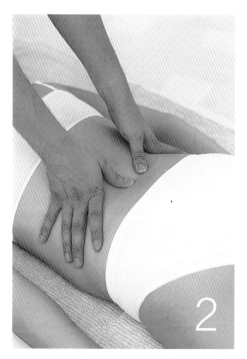

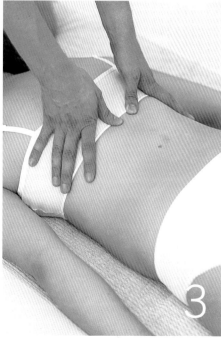

2

Move up to the sacral chakra in the abdomen and, working from the back, apply pressure with the pads of your thumbs, hold for three to five seconds and release. Repeat twice.

3

Move up to the solar plexus chakra and apply pressure with the pads of your thumbs, hold for three to five seconds and release. Repeat twice.

4

Move up to the throat chakra, which can be reached from the back of the neck. Apply pressure with the pads of your thumbs on either side of the vertebrae, hold for three to five seconds and release. Repeat twice.

5

The brow chakra can be balanced from the back of the head. Imagine a line from the brow through the skull and position the pads of your thumbs. Apply pressure, hold for three to five seconds and release. Repeat twice.

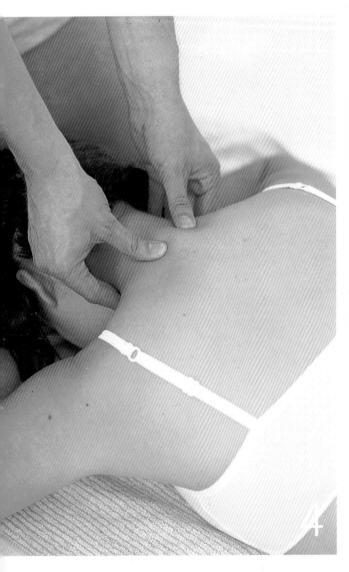

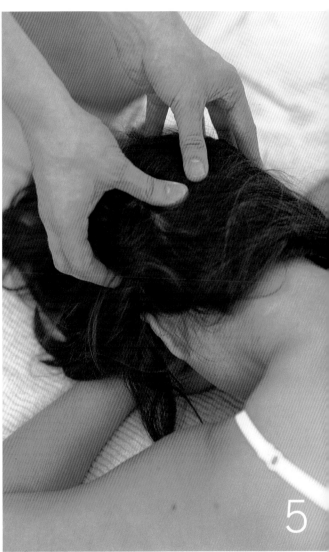

6

Finally, with the pads of your thumbs on the top of the head and fingers splayed to either side for support, apply pressure to the crown chakra, hold for three to five seconds and release. Repeat twice.

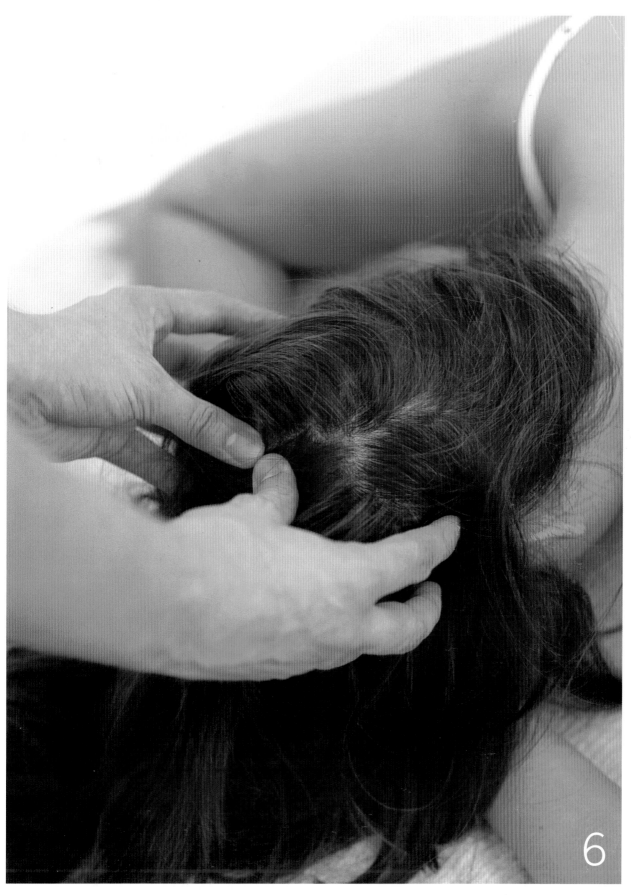

6

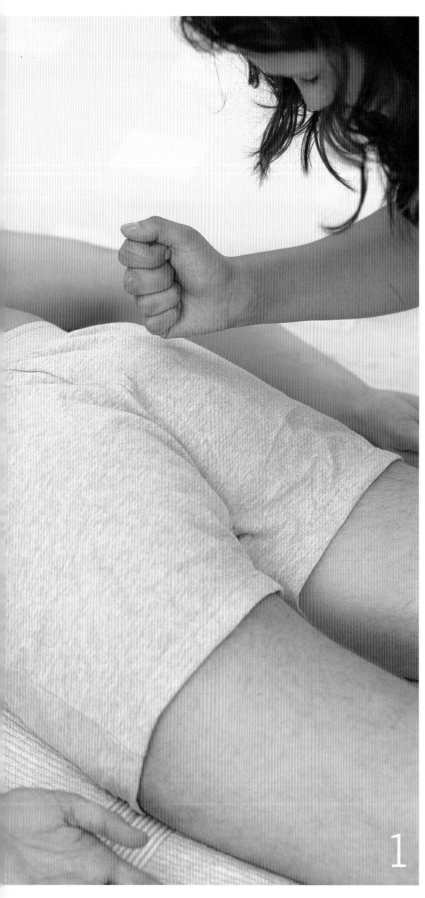

Lymphatic Massage

Applied in the mornings, lymphatic massage will give your immune system a boost and encourage the elimination of toxins and waste products, leaving you feeling more energetic and focused. Your lymphatic system plays an important part in maintaining correct fluid levels and defending the body against disease. It is a complicated filtering system made up of tiny vessels, but as the lymph glands have no muscles to help the flow and drainage, massage achieves this manually and so will speed up a sluggish system. Specially qualified therapists are trained to deal with medical oedema through this type of massage.

1

With your partner lying face down, make a fist with your right hand, swing out and punch the right buttock with your fist. Repeat five times. Repeat on the opposite side.

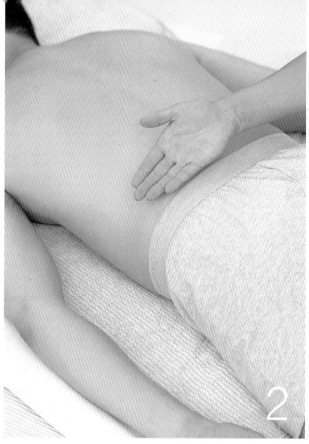

2

With a loose wrist, use the back of your hand to pat the kidneys very gently.

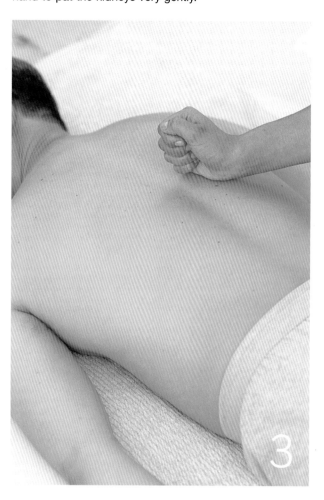

3

Make a fist with your hand, ask your partner to take a deep breath and thump the back below the shoulder blades on either side of the spine as they breathe out. Repeat five times.

4

Supporting your partner's arm at the wrist and upper arm, lift the arm upwards and then release it down, at the same time leaning back slightly to give a gentle pull. Repeat several times before moving to the opposite side.

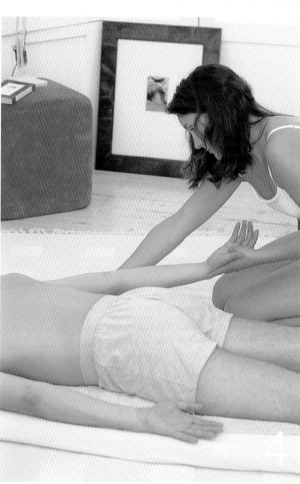

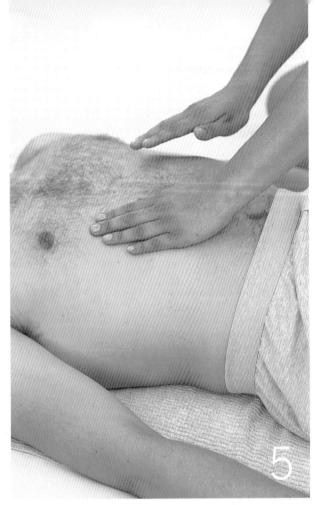

5

Ask your partner to turn face up and take a deep breath. Then, on the out breath, slap the ribcage lightly and quickly with the palms of both hands for 30 seconds.

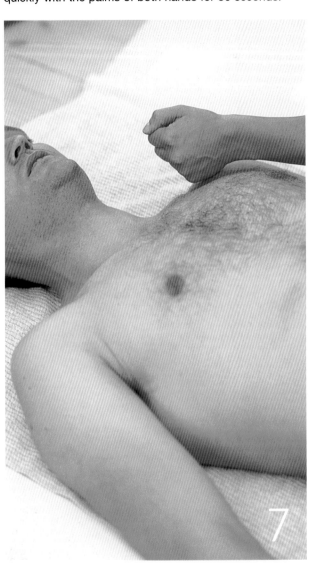

6

Moving your hands to underneath the ribcage, massage firmly from the sides of the body inwards towards the navel.

7

Ask your partner to take a deep breath and on the out breath, using your right hand in a fist, thump the area under the collarbone five times.

8

Repeat step 7 but use your left hand to clear the heart lymphatics on the right side of your partner's body.

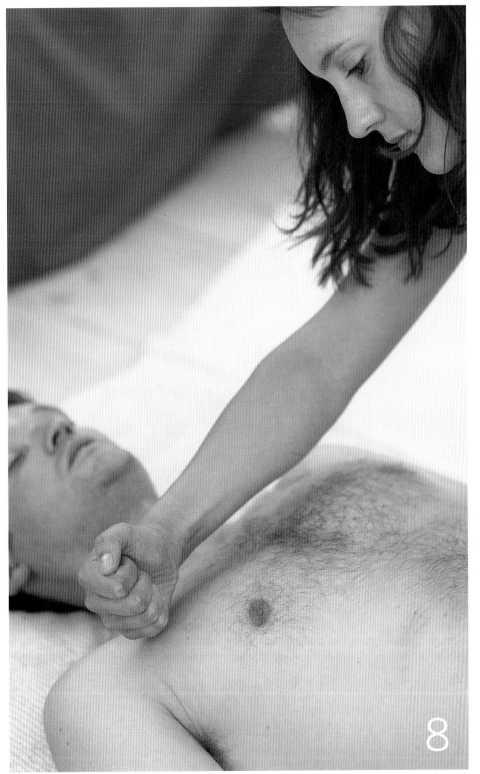

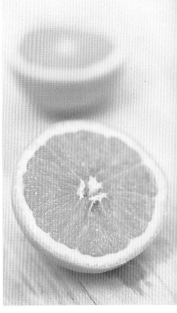

Tip

A glass of hot water and a slice of lemon, grapefruit or orange is a refreshing, cleansing and stimulating start to the day.

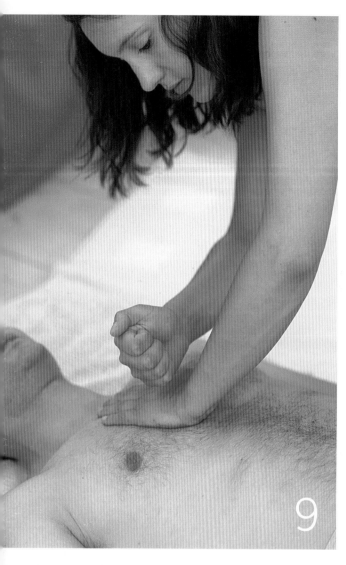

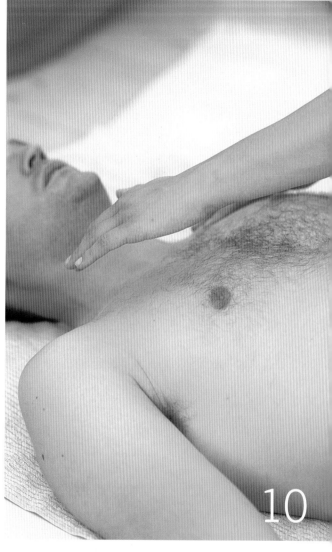

9

Place the flat of your hand on your partner's breast bone between the nipples, ask them to take a deep breath and, on the out breath, thump the top of your hand with the fist of the other hand five times.

10

Using the tips of your fingers in a tapping motion, work across the top of the chest very lightly.

11

Again using the tips of the fingers, tap down the sides of the neck simultaneously.

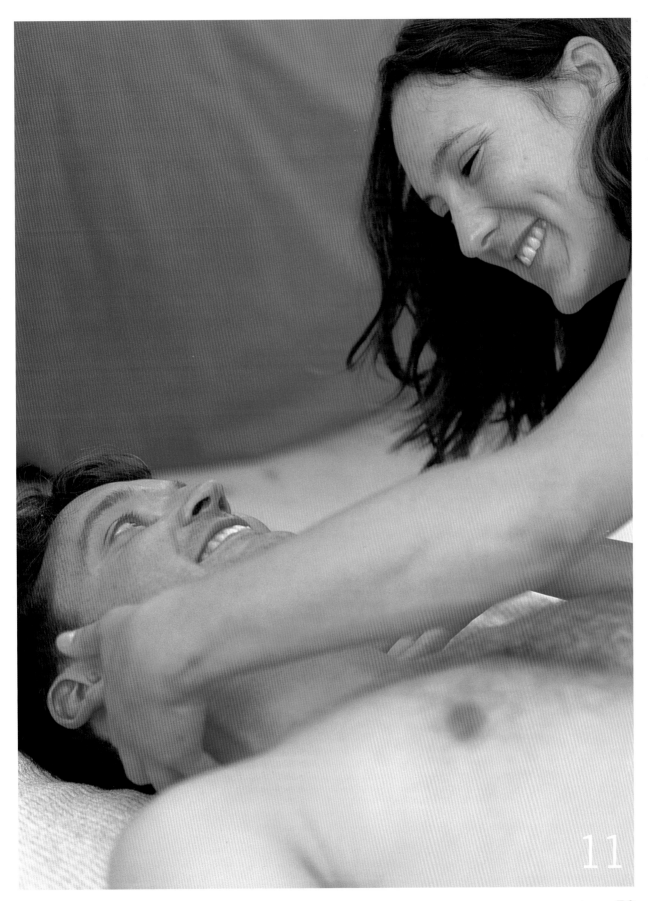

11

Massage Remedies

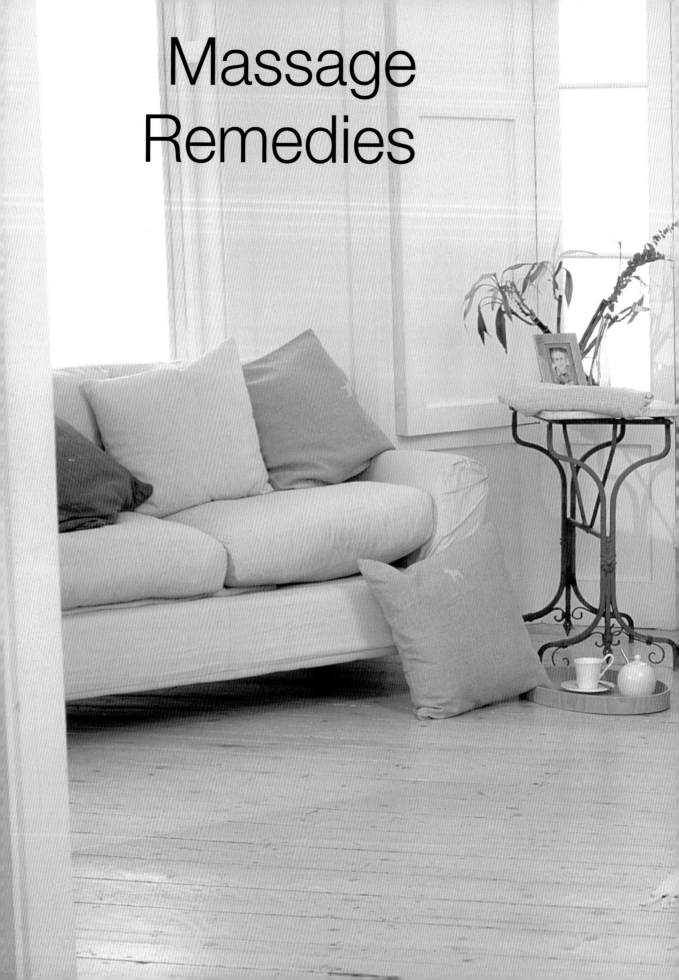

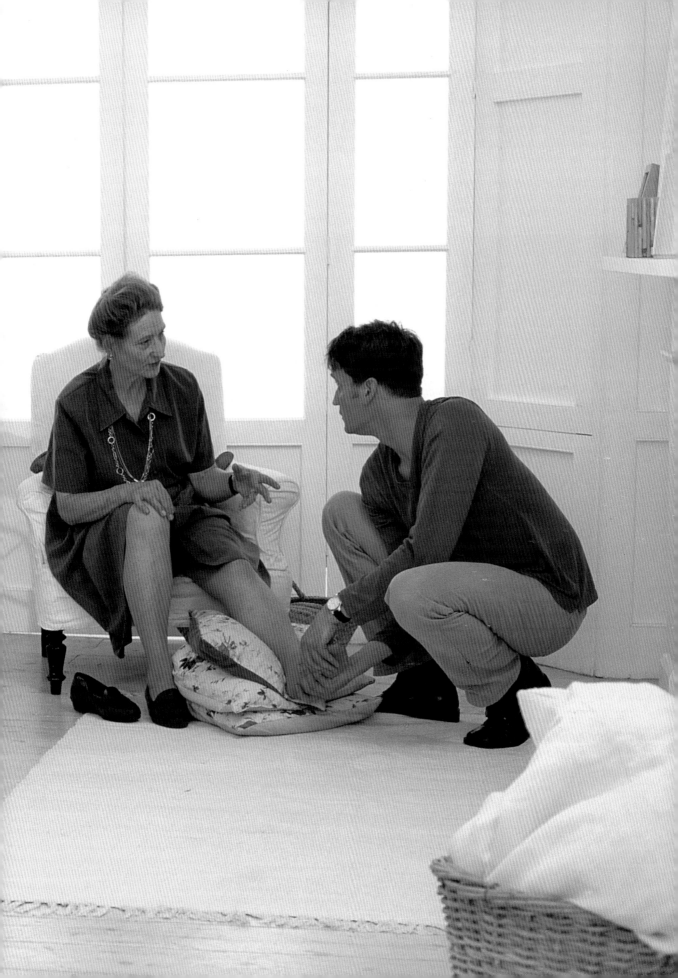

Sinusitis and Headaches

The most common complaints of the face and head area often respond very well to massage. The pain usually manifests itself at the base of the skull, the temples and forehead and at the top of the head, and is often caused by stress or bad posture. Migraine sufferers can also experience some relief, provided they feel comfortable enough to receive massage. The head provides a constant blood supply to the brain, and massage will help to stimulate this flow and prevent congestion. This is especially useful for people with poor circulation or hardening arteries.

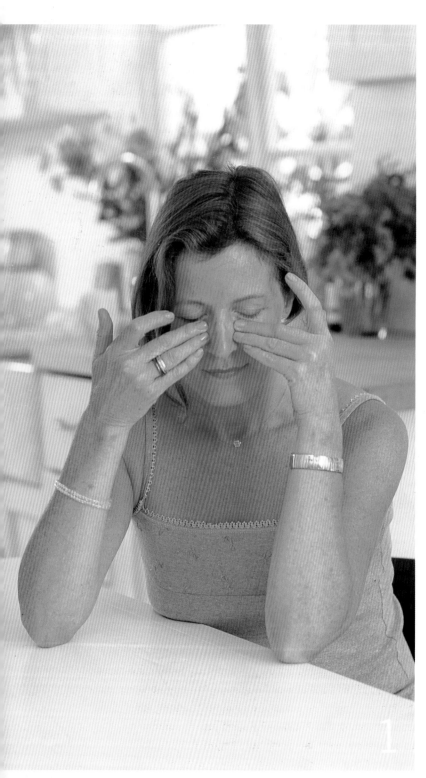

1 Sinusitis

The sinuses are hollow, air-filled cavities that drain into the nasal cavities. Congestion or inflammation of the sinuses results in a heavy, blocked-up feeling and pain in the face and head. Infection can be caused by such things as pollution or dirty water taken in while swimming. Self-massage is very effective because you can regulate the pressure according to the severity of the condition. Place your middle fingers on either side of your nose, breathe in and on the out breath glide your fingers down the sides of your nose to the nostrils and on to the cheeks, following the natural curve. Repeat several times. Palpating the areas at the beginning and end of this sequence will also help to drain the sinuses.

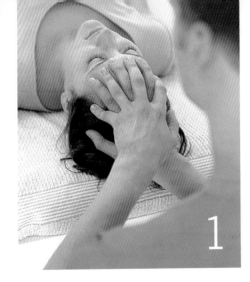

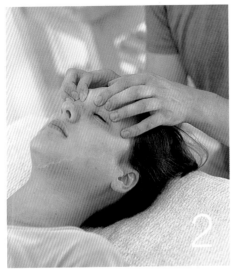

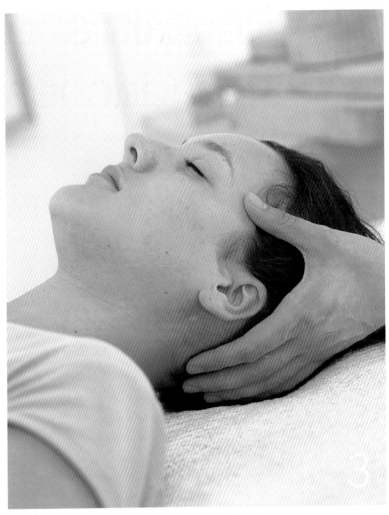

1 Headache

Place one hand with fingers spread slowly on your partner's head and forehead. Placing your other hand on top, slowly lean your weight into your hands until a comfortable pressure is achieved, hold for about 15 seconds and then release without losing contact. Repeat four to five times. This is a very subtle movement, and a headache in the forehead region can be relieved by this deep pressure.

2

Place the pads of your fingers just along the underside of the brow bones. Taking care not to apply too much pressure, because this area can be quite tender, hold for about 15 seconds and then release without losing contact. Repeat four to five times.

3

Move your hands to the sides of the head, with your thumbs positioned over the temples. Check with your partner that the pressure is comfortable and then rotate the pads of your thumbs slowly in a clockwise direction about 15 times – the slower the rotation, the more relaxing it will feel – then hold the pressure without rotating for about 15 seconds. Finish by bringing your hands down to cover both ears, wrapping your fingers underneath your ears and then drawing your fingers down and off.

Digestive Problems

Our digestive processes tend to reflect our state of mind. Stress can cause all sorts of conditions in this area, including irritable bowel syndrome (see pages 76–7), ulcers, indigestion, constipation or diarrhoea. This is because the blood supply is inhibited, and this, in turn, affects the way the digestive system absorbs and distributes nutrients. In addition, the muscle wall of the intestinal tract, which pushes the food through the body by contracting, cannot function properly.

The abdomen is the most exposed and unprotected area of the body, and is also the place in which we store our deepest emotions. In the East the *hara* (abdomen) is considered to house the body's vital energy. When massaging this area, be aware that your partner may feel vulnerable, so take some time to observe their breathing pattern and try to coordinate your strokes with this. You may find that even the lightest touch results in the instinctive self-protective action of a contraction of the abdominal muscles, so let your hands down gently. Before you start, pause for about 20 seconds to reassure your partner, lift off to apply oil and return gently, ready to start massaging.

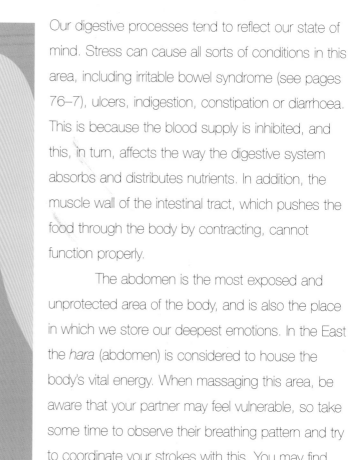

DIGESTIVE SYSTEM

❶ lungs
❷ liver
❸ stomach
❹ large intestine
❺ small intestine

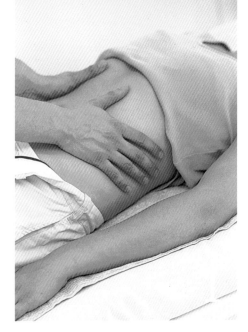

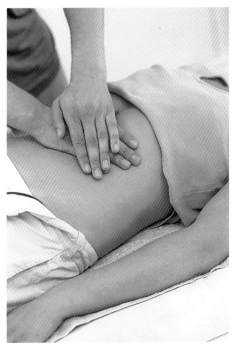

1

Using the effleurage stroke (see page 28), glide upwards to just under the breast area and then, with your hands on either side of the torso, slowly return to your starting position. Repeat five times in a flowing movement. This will calm and soothe the area and is particularly beneficial for abdominal bloating and indigestion.

2

Place one hand on top of the other and, making sure that your whole hand is in contact with your partner, work in a circular, clockwise movement from the solar plexus following the direction of the large intestine (see diagram, opposite top). Start with a large circle and continue, reducing the size of the circle but increasing the pressure, for a further four or five times. Remember to follow your partner's breath with your hands. You will find this movement helpful for relieving abdominal pain and constipation.

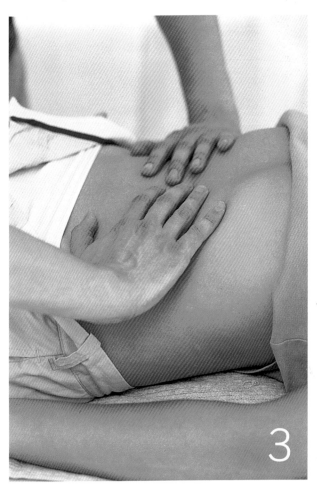

3

3

Always apply this stroke after you have relaxed the area with step 1. Using the flat of your hands and gentle pressure, on your partner's out breath draw your hands apart diagonally (left ribs to right hip, for example), working outwards in a sweeping action and remembering that this is more of a stretching movement than working deeply. Repeat in the other direction. This will help to release contracted muscle and so is excellent for menstrual cramping. Using a massage oil blended with chamomile, lavender or rose can provide additional relief.

Travel Sickness

Whatever mode of transport we use, and whether we are young or old, from time to time most of us suffer from travel sickness. More recently a condition called deep vein thrombosis (DVT) has been identified. It is linked with sitting inactively for long periods of time as in an aeroplane or car and involves the formation of a blood clot, usually in the calf area, which causes swelling and pain. A more serious consequence arises if this clot then travels around the body and ends up lodged in the lung. Massage can help, as it manually assists the blood flow through the deep veins and their valves in the legs onwards towards the heart, which would normally be achieved through movement and pressure.

TRAVEL REMEDIES

If you have to take a long trip, you can reduce the risk of DVT with a simple self-help programme.

- Keep your body hydrated by drinking plenty of water.
- Do not cross your legs, as this puts pressure on the blood vessels at the back.
- Make sure your socks and shoes are not constricting.
- Exercise your legs or, if possible, move about at regular intervals.
- If you suffer from varicose veins, clotting or have had a recent injury or surgery on your legs, consider wearing support hose.
- At intervals, apply some simple self-massage techniques.

1 Motion Sickness

Massaging this pressure point works in a similar way to the special wrist bands that you can purchase at most pharmacies and can relieve sickness. Place the pad of your thumb on the inside of your wrist in alignment with your first finger and apply pressure, using your fingers to support the back of the hand on which you are working. Repeat on the other hand.

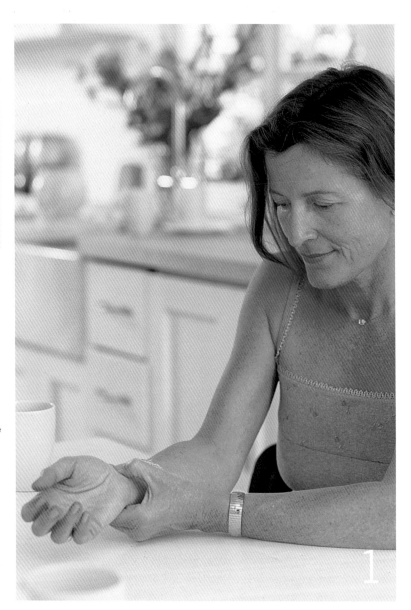

1

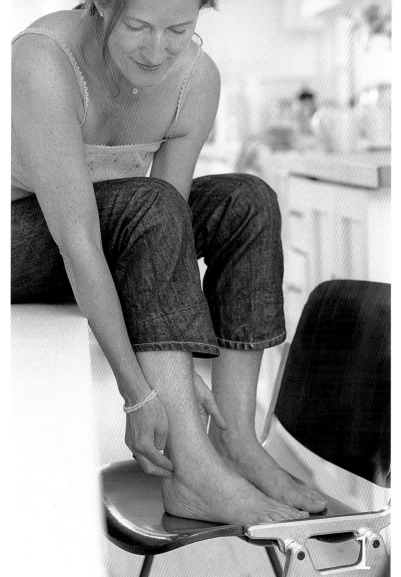

Deep Vein Thrombosis (DVT)

1

This is a simple technique which you can apply while you are sitting. With both hands working on one leg at a time, place the pads of your fingers on either side of your foot between the ankle and the heel. Working in a small circular movement, apply intermittent pressure as though you are manually pumping the area. Repeat on the other leg.

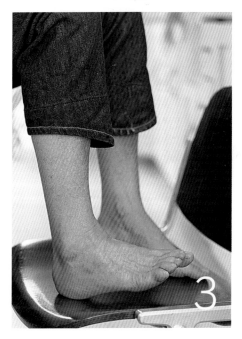

2

Using the knuckling stroke (see page 34), work both hands upwards from the ankle towards the knee area and return, with the pressure always on the upward stroke. You can apply this pressure in a straight or circular movement over the sides or back of the calves, but avoid any varicose veins. Repeat five times and then move to the other leg.

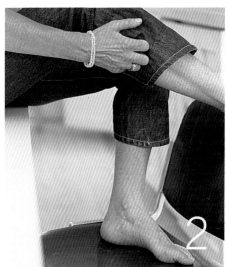

3

This simple pumping action is excellent for maintaining good blood flow. In a rocking movement and using both feet simultaneously, lift your heels and then tap your toes. You can move your feet in the same or alternate directions – you may enjoy doing this to music. Another variation on this exercise is to use an inflatable travelling neck pillow: place your feet on either side of the U shape and simply press down alternately, letting the air do the work.

Asthma

Characterized by intermittent breathlessness and wheezing, asthma is one of several common symptoms of respiratory stress. This distressing condition is much more common in our modern world, with possible causes including pollution, chemical allergies and irritants (such as smoking, and temperature changes). The difficulty in breathing is caused by spasm and inflammation of the bronchial tubes and their mucus lining and by a tightening of the chest muscle.

The frequency of attacks and the severity of the condition vary and are often related to emotional states such as stress and anxiety. This is where massage can play a very beneficial role in relaxing asthmatics, even being applied during an attack in a sitting position if the sufferers are comfortable with this. Remember to relax and warm up the area with gentle effleurage (see page 28) before applying the following specific movements.

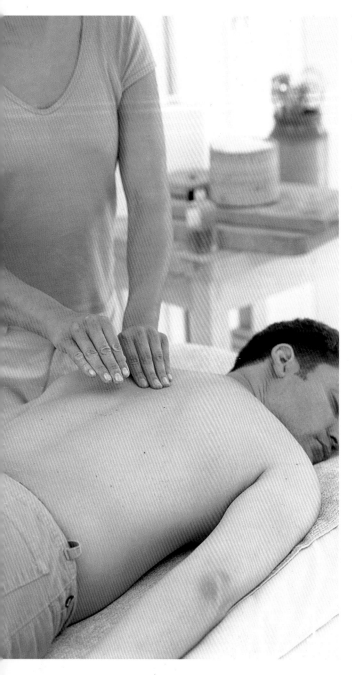

1

Using the cupping stroke (see page 33), work over the back area, avoiding the spine. Usually this movement is administered between attacks, when the sufferer is more comfortable, and helps to release any build-up of mucus.

SAFETY FIRST

Used on a regular basis, massage will help the asthma sufferer to maintain a relaxed state and so may contribute towards alleviating the condition. However, there are times when massage would not be appropriate:

- When there is a respiratory tract infection
- During an unrelenting attack
- If medication has not had any effect

Massage is not a substitute for medication and any changes in medication arising from the benefits of massage should be discussed with your doctor first.

2

Use the flicking stroke (see page 33) to apply friction to the the spaces between the ribs (intercostals). This will stimulate the local circulation, help to promote lymph flow and relax the muscles in this area.

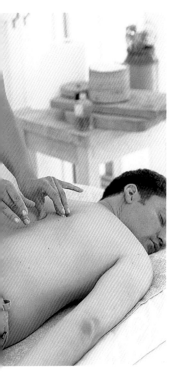
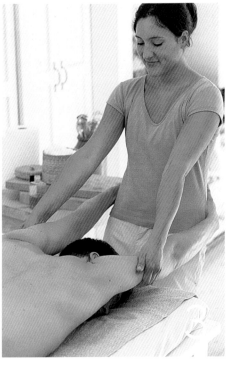

3

Passive movements help the expansion of the whole area, which is very useful if the sufferer is unable to exercise. Standing upright at your partner's head, place their hands around your lower back and, with your hands supporting their upper arms just above the elbows, ask them to take a deep breath. As they inhale, flex your knees and lean backwards. Maintain this stretch while they exhale and then ease off the traction, keeping hold of their arms, and straighten your knees, ready to repeat once.

4

For a bigger stretch, slide your hands down to your partner's forearms with their hands gripping yours and repeat step 3, stretching on the in breath and holding on exhalation.

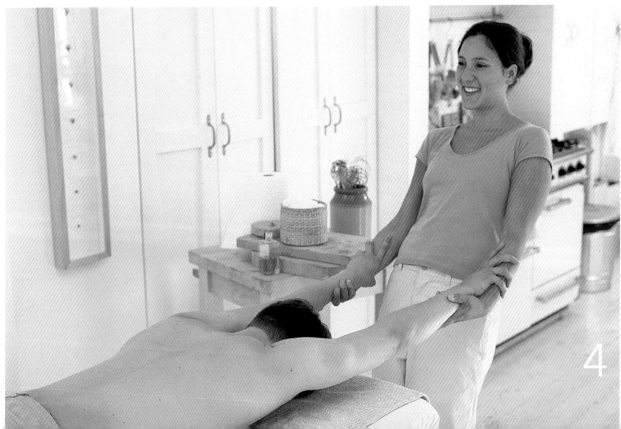

4

Menstruation and Menopause

Every month many women suffer from one or many of the effects of their hormonal cycle – including water retention, headaches, pelvic congestion resulting in back pain, cramping and nerve pain – the results of body imbalances caused by reduced progesterone and raised aldosterone levels. By inducing relaxation, massage can reduce the symptoms of premenstrual tension, such as tension, irritability, depression and crying spells. It can also release tightness in muscles and stimulate the blood and lymph flows, thereby helping in the elimination of toxins and excess fluid. It is, however, very important to work within the comfort level of your partner, as sometimes the body may feel too tense and sensitive for anything other than very light strokes.

During all the stages of the menopause, hormonal imbalance of a different kind is to blame for symptoms that include sweating, hot flushes, migraines and bloating. There are trigger points within the abdominal wall that, when treated, can bring relief – in contrast to abdominal massage, which can sometimes increase blood pressure and produce hot flushes. Gentle massage is ideal for reducing the musculoskeletal pain that is sometimes a characteristic of menopause.

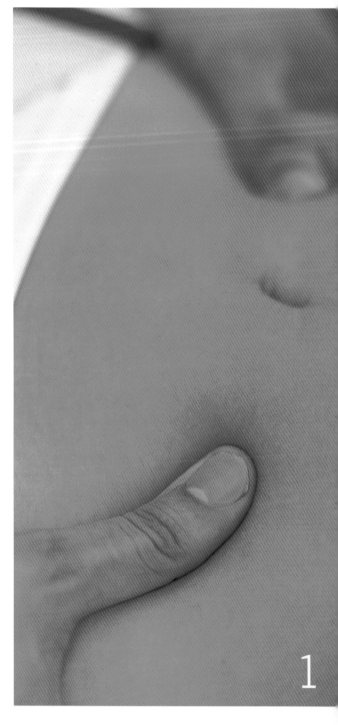

1

Place the pads of your thumbs about 7cm (3in) on either side of the navel and, using your body weight, lean in towards the navel and hold for five seconds. Repeat two or three times.

Herbal teas, which contain no caffeine, can be relaxing. Chamomile, fennel and meadowsweet can be especially helpful in relieving menstrual pain, cramps and menopausal problems.

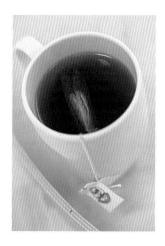

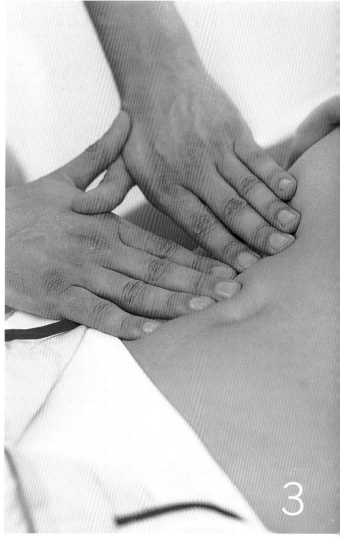

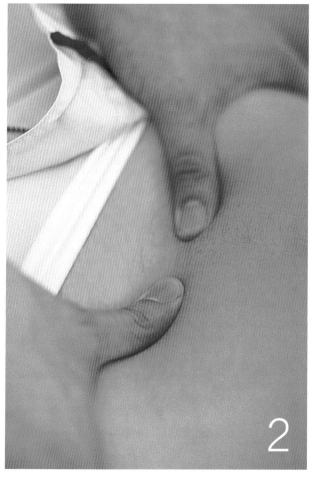

2

Move your thumbs close together and, using the pads, work as in step 1 downwards in a straight line, from just below the navel to end level with the hips, then work back up, finishing with your thumbs about 7cm (3in) on either side of the navel. This will relax stomach tension and reduce spasms and fatigue.

3

Using very light strokes and with your hands relaxed and close together, place them on the mid-abdomen, level with the navel, and effleurage (see page 28) gently in an arc towards the groin and return. Make sure that you massage both sides of the abdomen equally. As you become more experienced, you may wish to use an intermittent pressure technique instead of the gliding stroke. This time, use mostly the pads of your fingers and, instead of sliding, 'stretch' the tissues by alternately applying pressure and releasing as you move in an arc towards the groin. This is a very subtle movement and you should keep contact with your partner at all times. The technique works on the lymphatic flow and is especially effective in reducing water retention in the abdominal area.

Oedema

Derived from the Greek word meaning 'to swell', an oedema is simply an excess of fluid which can build up either inside or between cells. It can be situated in one specific area or may spread throughout the body. There are many causes, ranging from minor problems, such as premenstrual water retention, 'housemaid's knee', due to too much kneeling, and the effects of a hot climate, to more serious problems, including heart or kidney failure and lymphoedema (swelling of the lymph nodes). Massage can be very effective in dealing with some of the simpler problems, but treatment for more complex conditions requires professional training and, in some cases, a doctor's approval. The techniques shown here can also be adapted for self-massage.

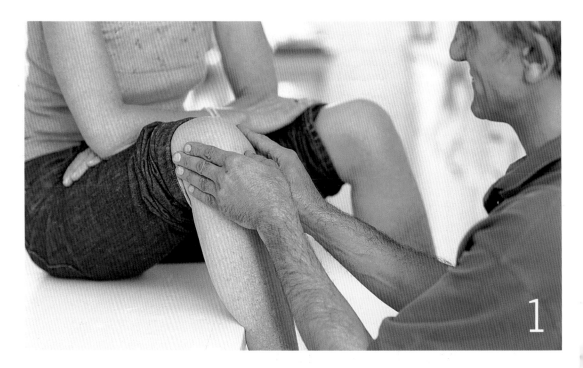

1

This technique is useful for dispelling 'water on the knee'. Working on one leg at a time and using the pads of your thumbs, work around the knee joint, starting at the top. Lean into the area surrounding the knee pad and move downwards on each side, applying pressure slowly and to a level that is comfortable for your partner. Direct each application of pressure inwards towards the centre and hold for five seconds before moving to the next position, until you have reached the area under the joint, completing the circle. Repeat on the other leg. To finish off, move to the feet and hold for 20 seconds to 'ground' your partner (see page 39).

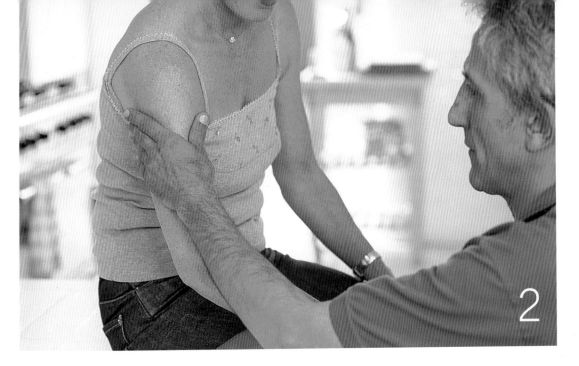

2

A build-up of fluid in the upper arm can result from over-exercising, hormonal changes during menstruation or poor lymph flow. Trained therapists use the technique of manual lymphatic drainage massage in place of the action of the body's lymph nodes if they are removed during a mastectomy. Support your partner's arm by holding the inside of their elbow and rest their forearm on yours. Using your other hand, lean into the outside of the upper arm and with your fingers and thumb squeeze over the muscle, slowly working upwards from the elbow to the shoulder. Return with flat-handed effleurage (see page 28) down the outside of the arm. Repeat up to five times before moving to the other arm. This movement is great for the circulation.

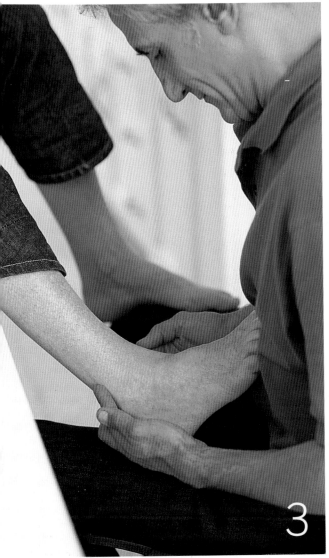

3

One of the most obvious areas of fluid build-up is around the feet and ankles. Long periods of walking on hot summer days, aeroplane cabin pressure or tight footwear will all result in a 'puffy' look, which can be eased by a simple 'drainage' massage. Making sure you support the foot, make small circular movements, always working around and not directly on the swelling. With your fingers under the heel for support, press your thumb pads simultaneously on both sides of the Achilles tendon and hold the pressure for five seconds.

Tired Feet

If you have a job that requires a great deal of standing or walking, there is nothing as revitalizing as a foot massage – it is also a great way to end a hard day's shopping! You may find it more soothing to use talcum powder instead of oil for this particular routine. It is a good one to teach youngsters to do on each other, on parents and on grandparents.

1

Place the flat of your hands on the top of the foot with one thumb on top of the other, ready to administer the effleurage stroke (see page 28). With powder to aid the glide and light pressure, on your out breath work up the front of the foot towards the lower leg. When you reach this point, glide back down on either side of the foot, leaning back to add a slight pull to the stroke. Repeat three to five times.

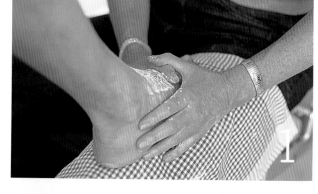

2

From a position that enables you to keep your arms straight, rest your thumbs and the heel of your hands on the top of the foot, with your fingers wrapped around the sides. Draw your thumbs across the foot in opposite directions, squeezing the foot firmly, and bring them down to join the rest of your hand in a movement that stretches and opens up the area.

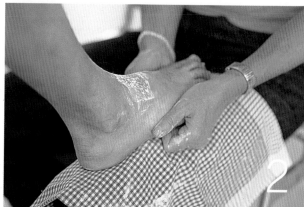

3

Make your hands into fists and apply the knuckling stroke (see page 34), circling all over the top and sides of the foot. Repeat several times. Now use the same strokes on the other foot.

This routine can be used alone or as a continuation of a leg massage; at the end, hold your partner's feet for 20 seconds to 'ground' them. In addition to revitalizing tired feet, this sequence will relax tension caused by high arches and even prevent winter chilblains, which are caused by poor circulation.

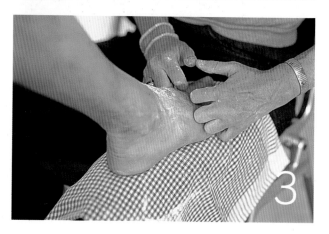

Calf Cramps

Calf cramps are muscle contractions that send the calf into spasm, and they may occur for no obvious reason. They can be alleviated with a simple kneading stroke (see page 31), which can be also be adapted for self-massage.

1

With fingers closed together, cup both hands around the back of the calf so that the tips of the fingers of each hand are facing each other along the midline of the calf muscle. Exert pressure with both hands simultaneously and roll the muscle using the kneading stroke, then release the pressure and repeat, slowly moving your hands up the whole length of the calf in order to reduce the muscle tension and relieve spasm.

2

Supporting the ankle with one hand, flex the foot to its point of resistance by pushing the toes and ball of the foot forward with the other hand. Reverse the action by pulling back the foot with one hand while pushing down on the heel with the other. This will release and stretch the calf muscle and also increase blood flow to the area, slowly reducing the cramping.

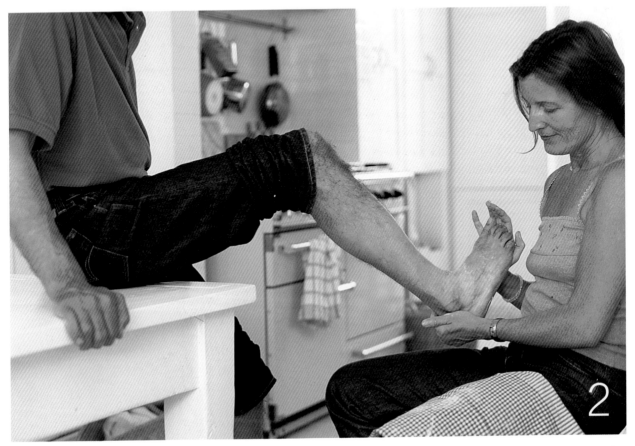

Irritable Bowel Syndrome (IBS)

This is a collective term for disorders of the bowel. Massage can often be very effective in relaxing the area and so reducing spasm of the involuntary muscles.

1

After warming up the area with gentle effleurage (see page 28), position yourself side-on to your partner and place your hands on opposite sides of the abdomen, cupped slightly over the sides of the torso. Using equal pressure and even weight on your palms and fingers, push one hand forward and the other back in a petrissage motion (see page 30), covering the whole of the abdomen from near side to far side.

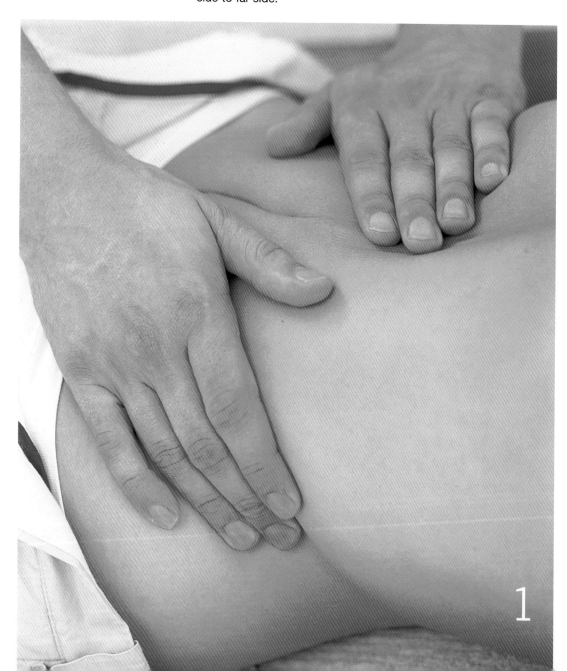

1

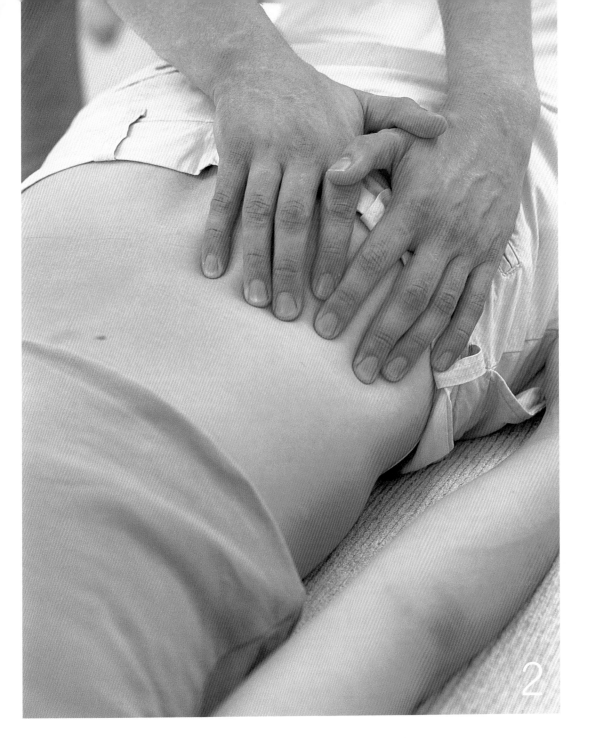

2

2

Place your hands just below the left side of your
partner's ribcage, with your fingers spread and facing
up towards their head. This is a vibrational technique:
as you apply pressure with the pads of your fingers,
make very small circular movements with each fingertip
simultaneously. This massages the descending colon and
helps to move its contents more smoothly along the
digestive tract.

Back Spasm

When a back is in spasm you cannot apply any deep strokes until the whole area has been warmed up and the muscles relaxed, so before a heavier stroking action a very light-pressured, criss-cross effleurage is used (see page 44). Once this has been completed you can continue with further treatment (see pages 104–9).

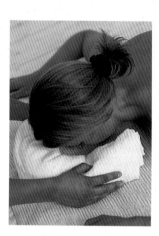

Tip

Folding a hand towel into a horseshoe shape creates a comfortable support for your partner's head while you are working on their back.

SELF-HELP BACK ROUTINE

The following easy routine helps the back as it relieves the pressure that we daily put on our discs in standing and sitting positions. It allows the back muscles to relax and in doing so lengthens the spine and allows the flow of fluid to the centre of the intervertebral discs, restoring their cushioning effect.

1 Wearing loose fitting clothing, lie down on the floor.

2 Make sure your head is well supported by a rolled-up towel or a pillow.

3 Bend your knees upwards so that your feet are flat on the floor, and hip width apart.

4 Rest your hands on your hips, arms on the floor.

5 Let the lower part of your back make contact with the floor.

6 Close your eyes and hold the position for a count of 20.

7 Bring your knees up to your chest, hug them, and hold for a count of 20.

8 Return to the starting position and repeat twice more.

SAFETY FIRST

Remember: always work on either side of the spine, never directly over it.

1

Facing your partner's side, place your hands on opposite sides of the lower back area on either side of the spine and apply the effleurage stroke, gliding your hands across the back in opposite directions. Continue working up the back area to the top and then repeat back down to where you started. Keep your rhythm slow, taking four to five seconds to glide from one side of the torso to the other. The aim is to achieve relaxation rather than stimulation.

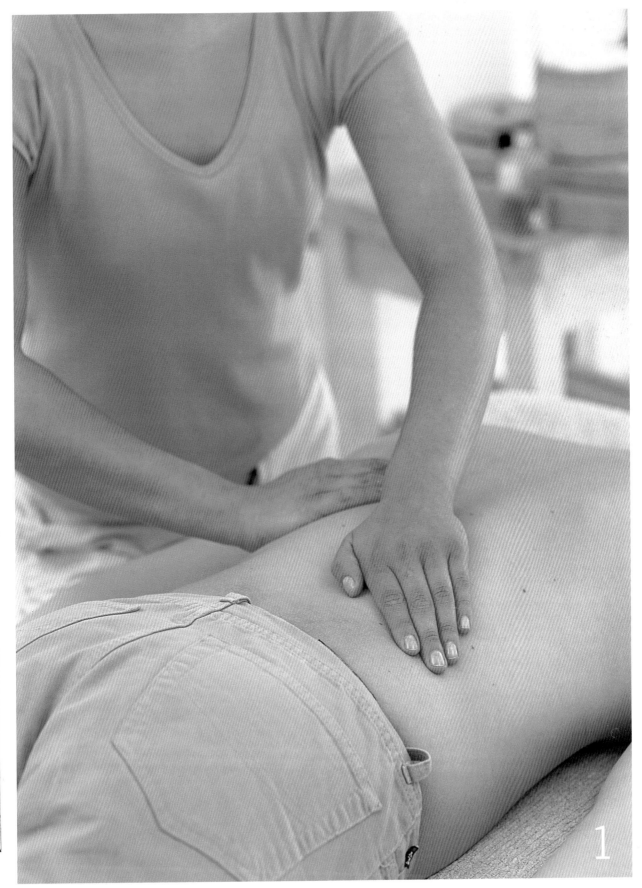

1

Pregnancy and Labour

Apart from the physical benefits, massage during this time is a way in which you can be of help and feel involved in your partner's pregnancy.

As the pregnancy progresses, your partner will have to adopt different positions in order to receive massage, and you will need to use lots of pillows to support her. Your partner may feel more comfortable straddling a straight-backed chair to receive back massage (see page 13), but by the fifth month lying sideways is advisable, with plenty of pillows placed around the stomach area and under the upper leg for support. This position is also useful for applying massage during labour.

SAFETY FIRST

Always observe the following safety precautions for massage during pregnancy:

- Do not massage during the first trimester.
- Avoid using deep pressure or vigorous strokes, especially on the abdomen, inner thigh and groin.
- Avoid applying pressure around and across the top of the ankles, as these points relate to the ovaries and the womb.
- Up to the 36th week of pregnancy, do not use essential oils in any form. Some oils are not suitable at any stage of pregnancy, so use a pre-mixed blend designed especially for the purpose or consult a qualified aromatherapist.

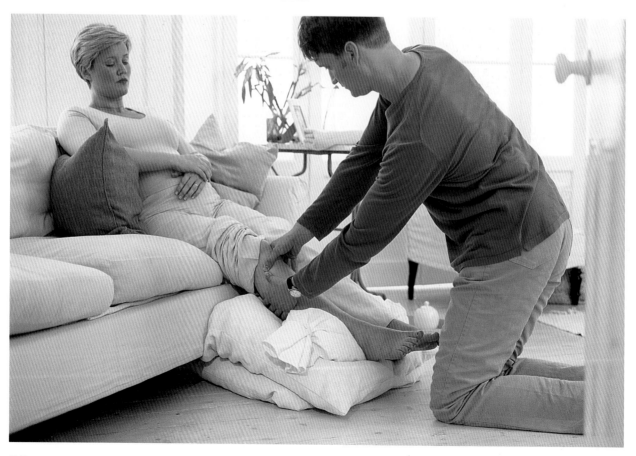

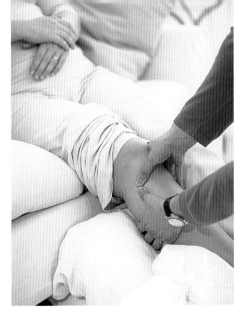

Legs and Ankles

Massage during pregnancy can be excellent, especially in the latter stages to reduce water retention and any circulatory problems, particularly those 'heavy leg' feelings.

1

Making sure that your partner's back and legs are well supported, place the pads of both thumbs at the top of the shin on the outer edge of one leg, where the bone widens towards the knee, and apply comfortable pressure three to five times. Working on this pressure point promotes energy and well-being and can also help with digestive problems.

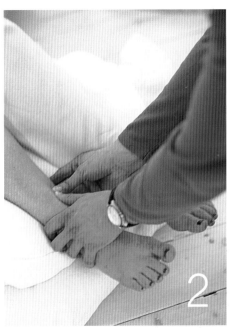

WHEN TO MASSAGE

FIRST TRIMESTER
Although body massage is not recommended,
a head or face massage can soothe away headaches or anxiety.

SECOND TRIMESTER
Indigestion and insomnia are common during this time, and
massage using very light, caring strokes can bring relief.

THIRD TRIMESTER
Concentrate on the back, neck, shoulders and particularly the
legs to relieve fatigue. The lower back and buttocks can be
massaged during labour to help the process along.

2

Moving down the leg, support your partner's foot with one hand and place the thumb pad of the other hand about four fingers' width above the inner ankle bone, once again applying comfortable pressure three to five times. This movement induces calm and relaxation.

3

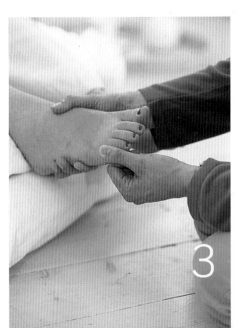

Finally, move down to the toes and, with one hand supporting the foot, take the small toe between your index finger and thumb and pull and squeeze in a downward movement, rotating the toe very slightly from the base to the tip. Apply to each toe.

Move to the other leg and repeat steps 1–3, finishing with a grounding hold (see page 39).

Neck and Lower Back

This area is often the weakest and most troublesome, and muscle tension in this area leads to shoulders being held unnaturally high by the end of the day.

1

You can work through your partner's clothes, but hand to skin would provide a more effective massage. Using the seated position described opposite, or with your partner lying on their side, warm your hands, apply oil or cream and then start at the lower back area using the flat of your hands in an effleurage stroke (see page 28). Glide up the back, with your hands on either side of the spine, across the shoulders and return, with your hands on either side of the torso, to the starting position. As with all back massage, the pressure should be on the upward stroke. Repeat three to five times. Next, work up the back, again using effleurage, but this time making small circles with your hands working in opposite directions, until you reach the shoulders and return as before. Repeat three to five times.

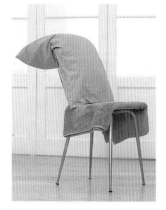

Tip

If your partner is pregnant she might find it more comfortable to straddle a straight-backed chair. Make sure there are pillows or cushions to lean against (see page 13).

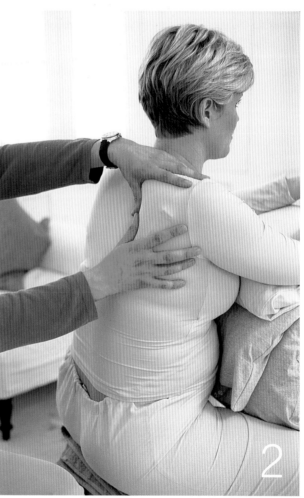

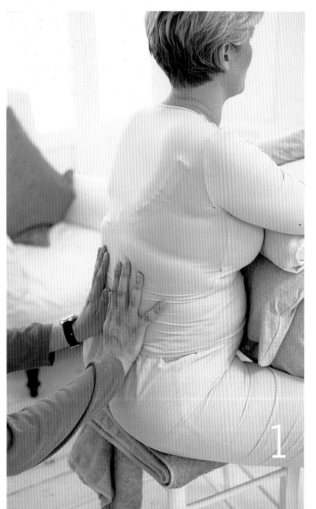

1

2

Working on one side at a time, glide across the shoulder blade. Then separate your hands, bringing one around the shoulder and the other around the armpit, pulling back gently as you return to your starting position. Repeat this movement three to five times and then move to the other side.

3

The next two strokes can be added to steps 1 and 2 in the same position or done on their own with your partner seated as shown. Start by making contact: bring your hands gently down to your partner and let them rest on the shoulders for about 30 seconds. Then, with your thumbs on the muscle at the back of the neck and your fingers over the front, begin to squeeze the shoulder muscles between the heel of your hands – not the thumbs – and your fingers, working from the muscle nearest to the neck outwards towards the tops of the arms and return. Repeat three to five times.

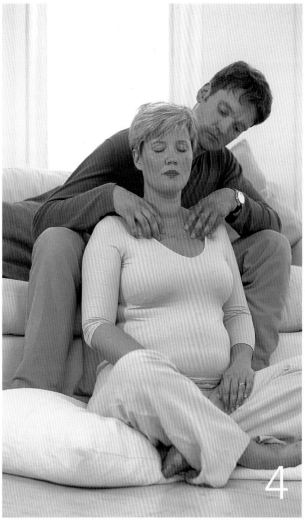

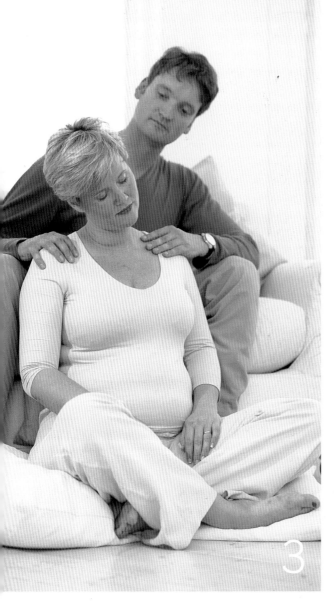

4

Using the effleurage stroke, but with your fingers splayed, work outwards from the breast bone (sternum) to the edge of the ribcage, using the pads of your fingers to massage the muscle between the line of the upper ribs. Repeat each stroke three to five times before moving to the next intercostal space, working from the top of the breast tissue upwards and asking your partner to take a few deep breaths between strokes. This will help to open up the whole area, which often feels pressured or restricted with the enlargement of the breast area as pregnancy progresses.

Baby Massage

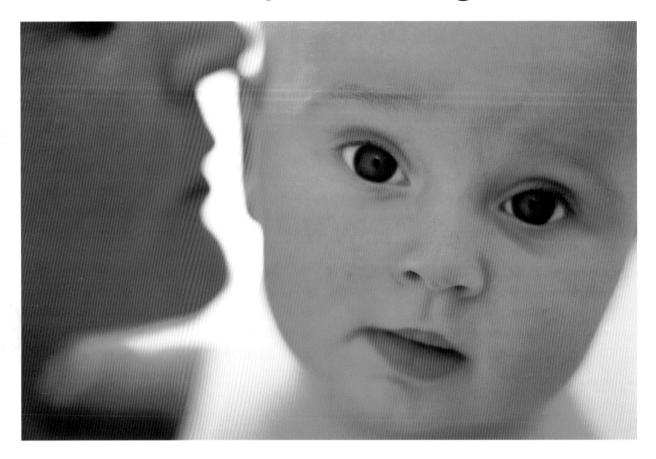

You are never too young to receive massage – in fact, paediatric research shows that massage helps babies to progress far more rapidly in growth and communication. They also sleep and feed better with regular stroking and stretching. In the first few months, common complaints such as colic or constipation can be relieved and good muscle tone can be encouraged. Massage is also a very powerful tool of communication and strengthens the bond between parent and baby. You may find that massaging a baby is quite challenging as they are not the most passive of partners, often wanting to take an active part in the procedure! After a while, however, they will begin to relax and enjoy the experience, and you will become more confident.

Once you have made the necessary preparations (see opposite) and are ready to start the massage, remember always to 'listen' to your baby. You should never proceed without full cooperation, so show lots of love and affection before and during the massage and maintain eye contact as much as possible. If the baby becomes distressed, stop and give comfort.

SAFETY FIRST

Always observe the following safety precautions
when massaging a baby:

- Wait until after the baby's full
health assessment at four to
six weeks of age before
giving a full massage
sequence. Before this, use
light stroking only.
- Do not massage if there is a
problem of unstable joints or
brittle bones.
- Be extra careful to avoid
massaging directly on
the spine.

- Wait for a week following
any vaccination before
massaging.
- Do not massage if the baby
has an infection, skin rash or
is being given any form of
medication.
- Wait for at least 1½ hours
following the baby's last
feed before massaging.
- For premature babies,
administer only light stroking
rather than a full massage.

Preparation

- Make sure the environment is very warm,
as babies lose body heat much more
quickly than adults.
- Use a changing mat covered with a clean
towel or work with your baby on your
knees or lap.
- Keep a towel close by in case of
'accidents'.
- Use a simple vegetable oil such as
sunflower, a pre-blended oil made
specifically for babies or talcum powder.
- Make sure your hands are warm and free
of any jewellry.

Full Body Massage

Lay your baby down in a comfortable position
for you both and starting with the chest follow
steps 1–11 for a full massage sequence
paying attention to our safety precautions.

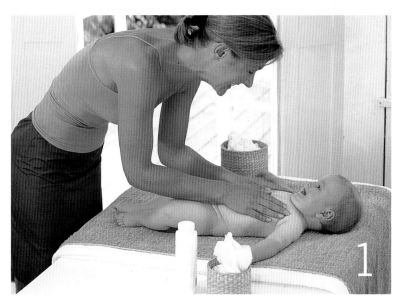

1

Place both hands together on the
centre of the chest area and gently
push outwards using a firm, assured
touch to avoid tickling, then bring
back to the centre in a heart-shaped
movement.

2

Rest your hands gently on the
centre and use an effleurage
stroke (see page 28) upwards
and outwards towards the
shoulders, then return down the
sides of the torso, back to the
starting point.

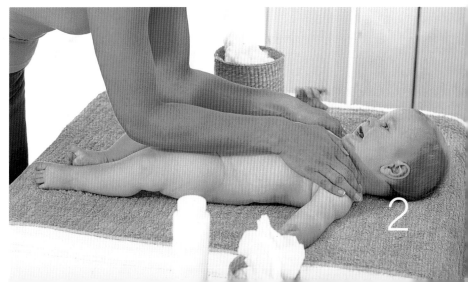

3

Working on one arm at a time, hold your baby's upper arm between your thumb and fingers, using your other hand to support the lower arm, and with the pad of your thumb massage in circles between the elbow and armpit.

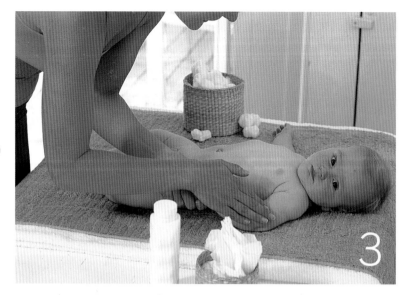

4

Move to the lower arm and repeat the circling movement down to the palms of the hands.

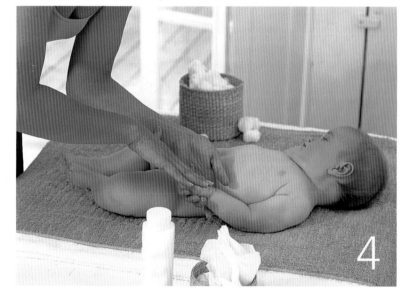

5

Using your thumb and index finger, massage the fingers one at a time until you have completed the whole hand.

   Move to the other arm and repeat steps 1–3.

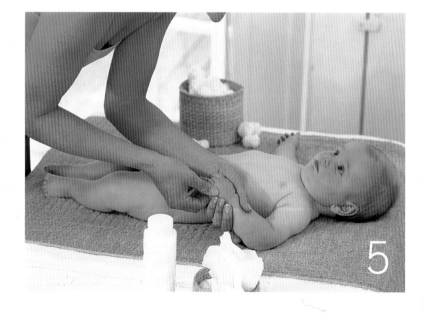

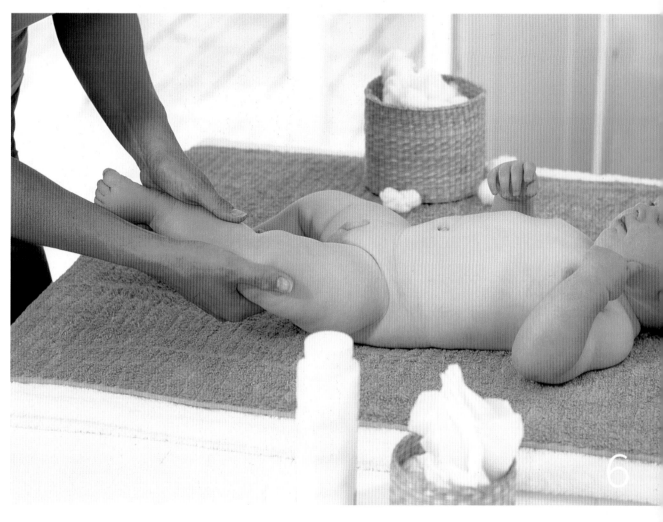

6

The same technique is used for the legs as for the arms, but first of all use the effleurage stroke (see page 28) to apply oil or cream. Working on one leg at a time, use one hand to support the lower leg and with the other use the pads of your thumbs to circle from the knee to the hip and then the groin. Repeat from the ankle to the knee.

7

To massage the feet, repeat the technique used for the hands and fingers (see page 86, step 3), using your index finger and thumb.

Move to the other leg and repeat steps 1 and 2.

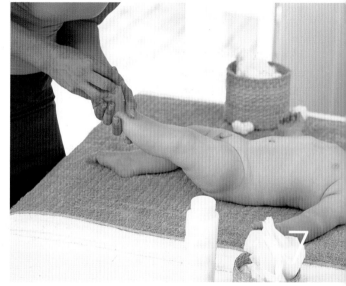

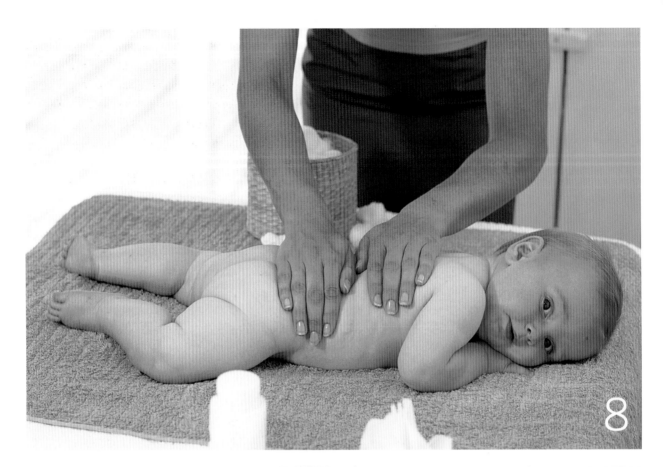

8

Place one hand on each side of your baby's back and, using the wringing stroke (see page 31), work from the bottom up to the shoulders and then down again. Keep your rhythm smooth and steady – your baby will find this very relaxing as it calms the spinal nerves.

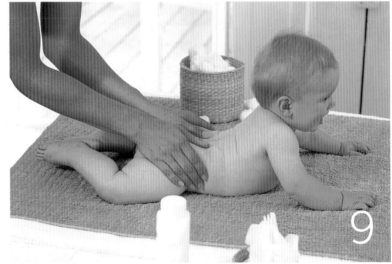

9

Place one hand on each buttock and, using the pads of your thumbs, massage in circles. Work upwards towards the sacrum and waist until you have covered the whole of the area.

10

Using long, sweeping effleurage strokes (see page 28), work up the whole of the back, across the shoulders and return down the sides of the torso to the starting position.

11

Using tiny thumb circles, work up first the left and then the right side of the spine, returning with a sweeping stroke over the shoulder and down the side of the torso. Finish off by stroking the whole of the back, connecting the back and legs.

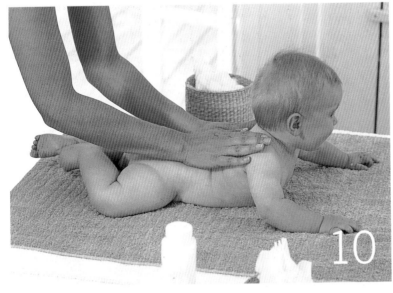

Massage benefits

All the strokes for baby massage can be repeated three or four times, but this will depend on the baby's response and how they adjust to the positions. Ideally, a massage should last for about ten minutes, but it may take a while to find a routine the baby enjoys. Observe the baby's responses and stop when these indicate they have had enough. Your baby may feel thirsty afterwards as the massage encourages the elimination of toxins. Try to do a sequence every day at a time when your baby is receptive and neither tired nor hungry – you will both benefit from the results.

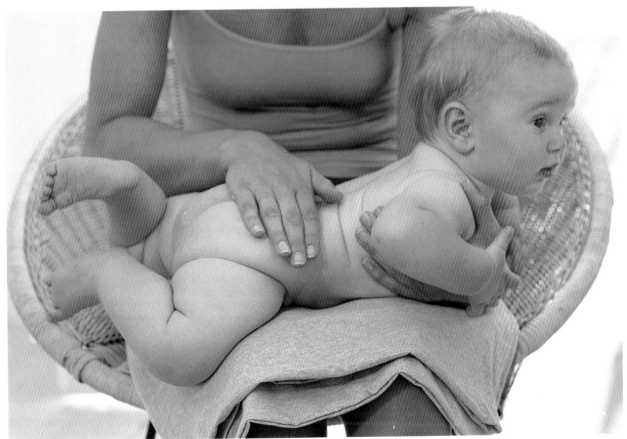

Treating Older People

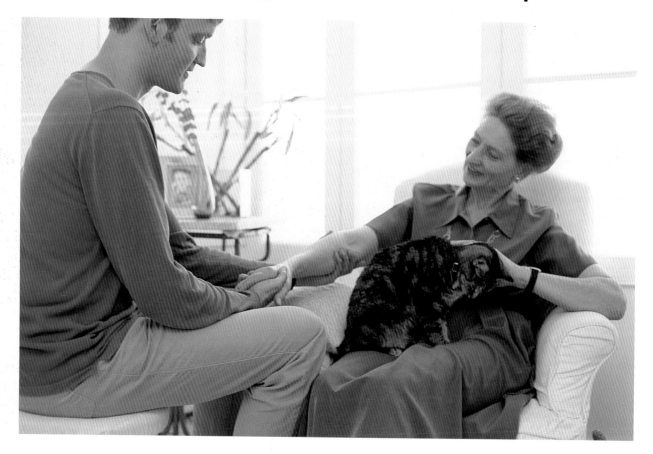

No matter how old we are, touch is essential for well-being on both a physical and an emotional level, but as people get older, some may feel they become 'invisible', and nurturing diminishes. Massage can play a major part in keeping the elderly healthy and supple, bringing the 'young' person inside nearer to the surface and enhancing their quality of life. It is also a great way to bridge that age gap: encourage grandchildren to massage their grandparents, or children their parents, for example.

Some common ailments at this time of life are joint pain, poor circulation and muscular stiffness, and because of these it will not always be comfortable to lie on the floor or a massage table. The routines shown here can be given in a seated position, working through the clothing. Make sure you use a good quality oil, such as almond, if you choose to work directly on the skin, which becomes thinner and drier with age. You may also need to reduce the pressure applied – work with your partner to find a comfortable level. If they suffer from arthritis, work very carefully and do not massage at times of inflammation.

Arms and Hands

Older people often have poor circulation, resulting in stiffness in their hands and feet. Massage increases the blood supply to these areas and helps mobilize joints – this technique can be adapted for self-massage.

1

Make sure you are both sitting in a comfortable position in a warm environment. Working on one arm at a time, support your partner's hand and wrist from underneath and work with your other hand. You may wish to start and finish this sequence with flat-handed effleurage (see page 28): glide up the forearm and return by twisting your hand around at the elbow and gliding the fingers down the underside of the arm to the wrist. This will warm and oil the area and also relax your partner. With your partner's arm well supported, place your hand on the outside of the arm and, using the petrissage stroke (see page 30), work up the forearm, squeezing the muscle between the heel of your hand and your fingers. Ease off the pressure over the joint area, then continue along the upper arm to the shoulder and return to the wrist.

2

Continue in the same position and, starting just above the wrist with your thumb on the top of the forearm, glide the thumb pad up to the elbow, twist your hand around and return with the fingers gliding down the underneath of the arm back to the wrist. Repeat each movement three to five times.

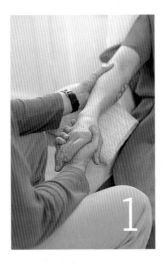

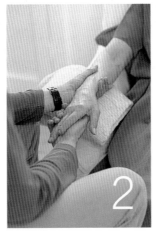

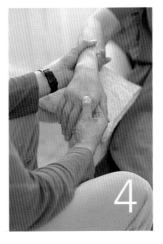

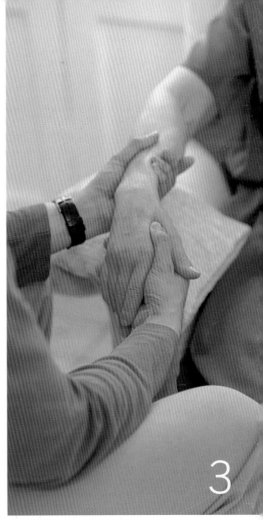

3

Still supporting the arm, place your thumb in the web of your partner's hand between the thumb and first finger and apply pressure inwards for about five seconds. This is a pressure point called the 'Great Eliminator' and helps to dispel headaches and colds and aid digestion.

4

Work over the entire back of the hand with the thumb pads in a circling stroke, making sure that the hand and wrist are well supported. This is a simple move that your partner can learn to do for themselves daily.

Move to the other arm and repeat steps 1–4.

Feet and Legs

Increasing the blood flow to this area will combat conditions like winter chilblains, reduce the water retention that leads to swollen ankles and generally relax the feet and ankles. Once again, these moves can be applied either with or without socks or stockings; however, there is nothing as luxurious as having your feet massaged with wonderful essential oils such as lavender or chamomile.

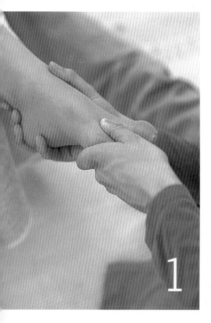

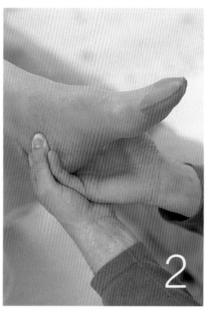

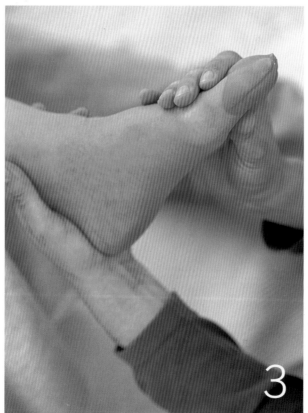

1

Make sure that you are both in a comfortable working position and that the leg you are working on is well supported. With one hand placed under and around the ankle to take the weight of the foot, using the thumb pads in a circling stroke, work over the whole of the top of the foot. As a variation on this, use the circular knuckling stroke (see page 34).

2

Press your thumb pad into the hollow between the ankle bone and the Achilles tendon, slightly to the front and outside of the ankle. Hold for three to five seconds, then release and repeat two or three times. Working on this pressure point can reduce water retention and can also relieve lower back pain.

3

Place your hand on the top of the foot with your thumb underneath and, using thumb circling and starting at the heel and ending at the ball of the foot, work across the whole of the sole, using firm, even pressure so that you do not tickle your partner. Support the heel and ankle with the other hand. This area of the foot contains thousands of nerve endings and reflex connections, and so is ideal to massage if a whole body treatment is not possible.

Move to the other foot and repeat steps 1–3.

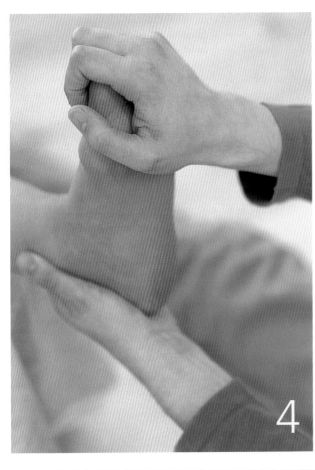

4

Flexing the feet helps to make joints more mobile and stretches the hamstrings at the back of the legs. Facing along your partner's body, hold the ankle firmly with one hand and with the other push on the toes and ball of the foot until you reach a resistance point that is comfortable for your partner. Hold for five to ten seconds and release.

5

Place your hand on the top of the foot and gradually pull downwards while pushing the heel with your other hand to a comfortable point of resistance. Again hold for five to ten seconds and release. This stretches the front of the leg and the top of the foot.

You can repeat these two moves three to five times each, then finish off with a gentle stroking movement downwards from the ankle to the toes, before moving to the other leg and foot.

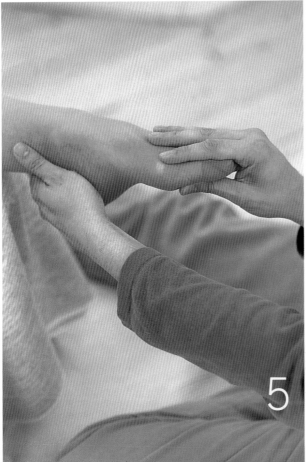

SAFETY FIRST

Always observe the following safety precautions when flexing the feet:

- Work gradually and make sure you stay within your partner's physical limitations.
- Keep the leg flat, so that any pressure applied is in alignment with the knee.
- Stop at once if your partner experiences any sharp pain – particularly in the back of the leg, which could indicate lower back problems or even sciatica.

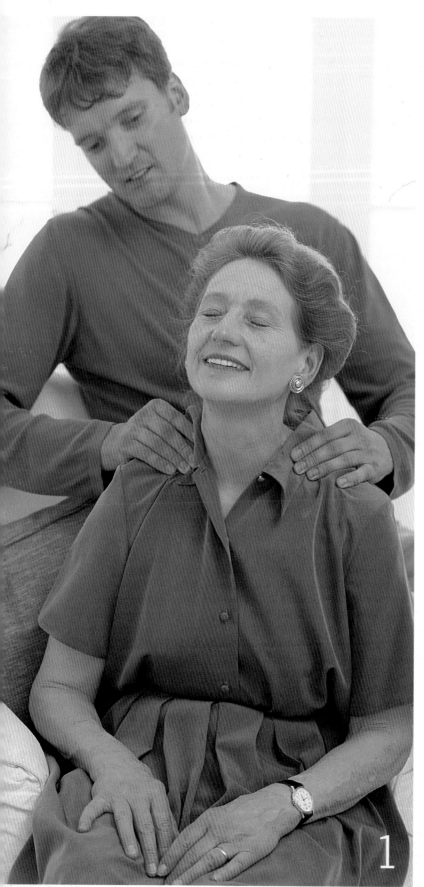

Neck and Shoulders

This area is often the weakest part of the body and is also where we store the most tension. Lack of exercise and a sedentary lifestyle will lead to reduced mobility here. Sometimes, the ageing process leads to stiffness in the neck and shoulders due to degeneration processes. A muscle called the trapezius dominates this whole area, and restriction or contraction here will result in discomfort, so the aim is to keep this muscle relaxed with the aid of massage. This routine is done through the clothes without the use of oil and so is easy to do at any time, in any place, as a quick pick-me-up or as a longer, relaxing experience.

1

Stand or sit behind your partner at a height comfortable to you both. Make contact by bringing your hands slowly downwards and gently resting one on each shoulder. Keep this contact and encourage your partner to close their eyes, let go of all thoughts and relax – this will make the muscle easier to work with. You will also be able to sense just how much tension your partner has stored in this area. Your fingers should be forward, over the tops of the shoulders, with the heel of your hand and your thumbs behind. Using a petrissage stroke (see page 30), squeeze the muscle gently between the heel of your hand and your fingers, working along the top of the shoulder blade and increasing the pressure and depth when required. This is an almost instinctive stroke that we often do with no instruction.

2

Carry the petrissage stroke downwards over the shoulder to the upper arm, ending just above the elbow, and return – the movement will feel uncompleted to your partner if you massage only to the edge of the shoulder.

3

With your hands cupped behind the neck and using the pads of all your fingers, work in very tiny circles up towards the base of the skull on either side of the neck vertebrae, stretching as you go. Place your fingertips on the ridge at the base of the skull and, making sure your fingers are not on the neck or head, apply pressure and hold for five to ten seconds, then rotate the pads of your fingers very slowly three to five times. If you want to finish this sequence here, stroke the fingers of alternate hands through your partner's hair to the top of the head in a combing action, then place your hands one on top of the other, on the top of the forehead and hold for ten seconds.

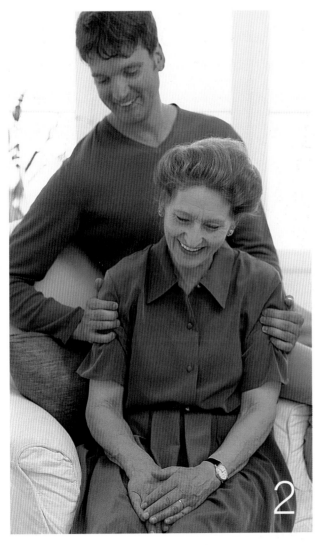

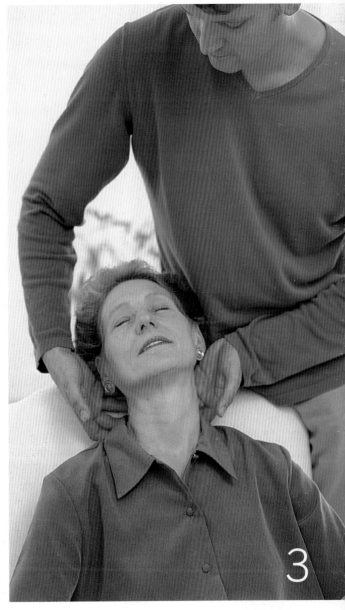

Tip

A warm bath with epsom or aromatherapy salts will help to warm the muscles before a massage or relax them before bed.

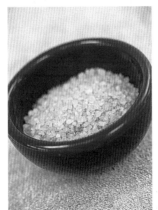

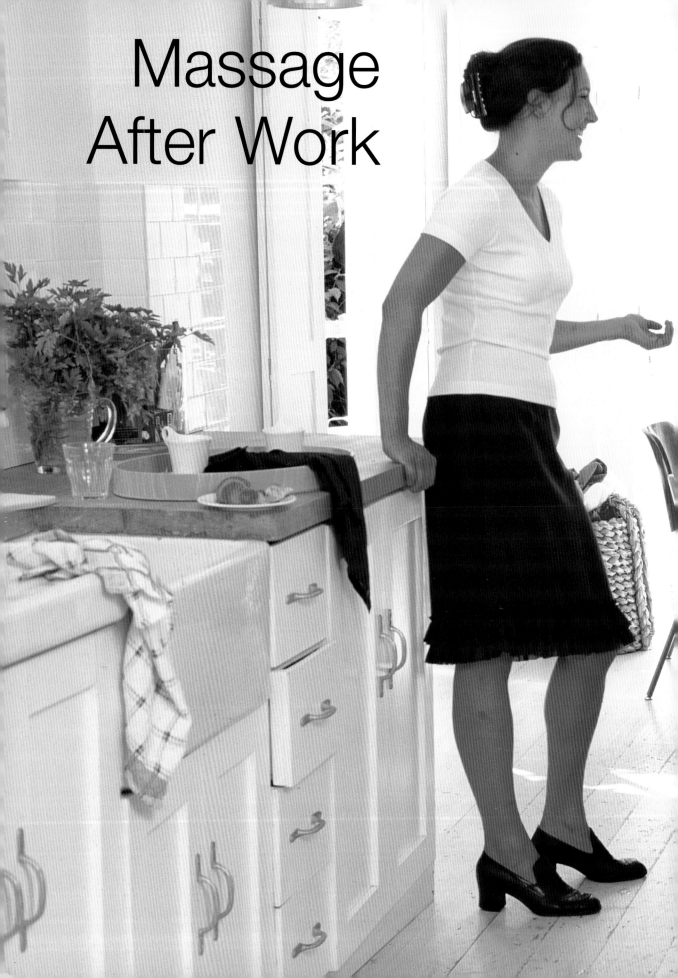

Massage
After Work

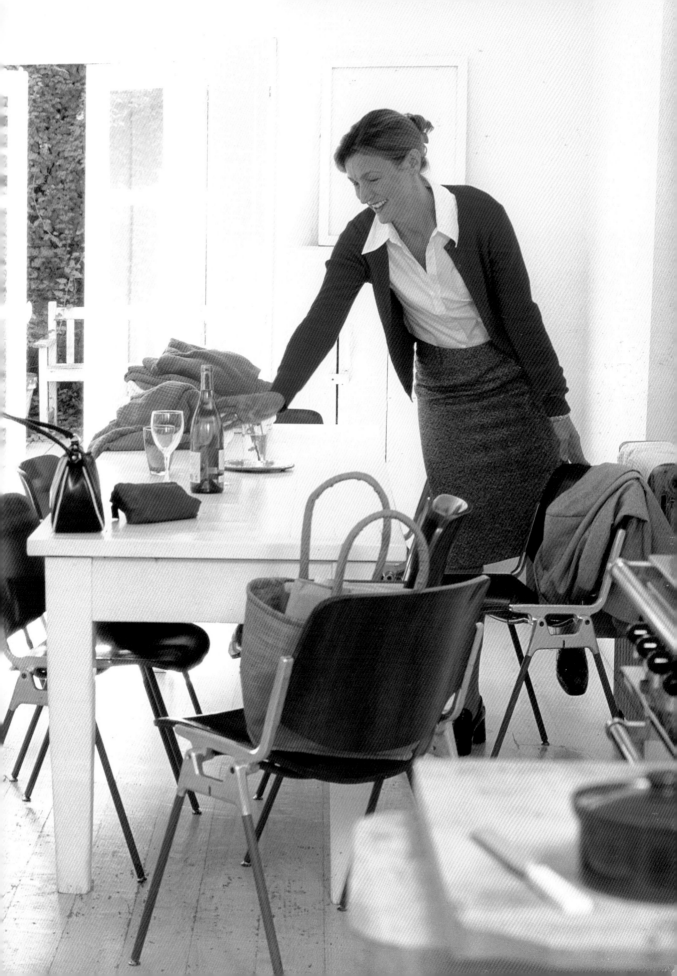

Repetitive Strain Injury (RSI)

RSI is finally being recognized as a real health problem relating to the workplace – but what exactly is it? It is actually a collective term used for carpel tunnel syndrome, non-specific arm pain, occupational overuse and work-caused disorders of the upper arm. Although we often associate it with the strain of using a keyboard, it can be caused by any repetitive action, and it affects musicians, checkout operators and assembly-line workers alike. Even housework or a hobby involving a specific physical movement can be a cause.

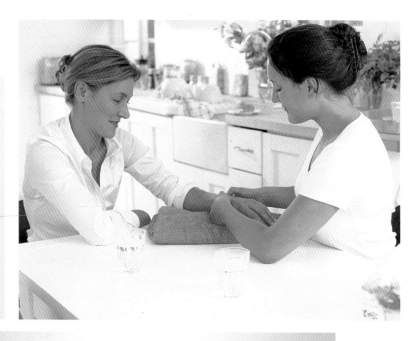

CHECK YOUR SYMPTOMS

The following are all symptoms of RSI:

- Weakness or loss of function in the muscles and joints of the hands, arms, shoulders or neck.
- Tingling, numbness or cold feelings in the hands and fingers.
- Swelling or a sense of swelling.
- Persistent pain even after resting.

HOW TO PREVENT RSI

Follow these guidelines to help you avoid RSI:
- Take regular breaks to avoid long periods of continuous, repetitive movement.
- Make sure your work station is ergonomically sound.
- Concentrate on your posture. For desk work, make sure your wrists are kept straight and your forearms are supported.
- Practise stretching exercises for the hands, neck and shoulders at regular intervals.

If you think you have symptoms of RSI, do not ignore them or camouflage them with painkillers, as only body maintainence will bring relief. Acupuncture, the Alexander Technique for posture and massage can all play a part in the prevention of RSI.

Hands and Wrists

The simple routine shown here can be done any time, anywhere. A good time is after work, perhaps while you and your partner are catching up on the day's events. You only need to use a little oil or, if you prefer, a favourite hand cream, which will rehydrate the skin at the same time.

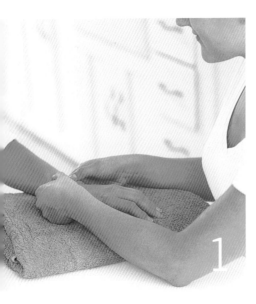

1

Using the pads of your thumbs and rotating them alternately in opposite directions, work in between and over the bony area of the wrist.

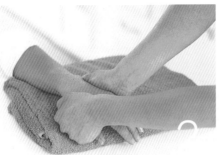

2

Starting with the heel of your hands on the centre back of your partner's hand, apply pressure and glide them in opposite directions across to the edge, where your fingers are wrapped around your partner's hand. This will really stretch and open up the area. Repeat this step three to five times.

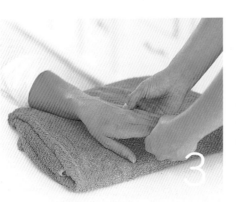

3

Holding your partner's hand, place your thumb pad just above the web between the third and fourth fingers, then apply pressure and glide up towards the wrist, following the hollow channel between the knuckles. Move to the web between the second and third fingers and repeat the movement, continuing in this way until you have worked all four areas.

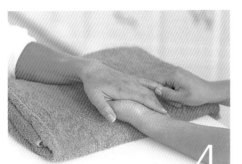

4

Supporting your partner's hand in a flat, handshake-type clasp, take the little finger at the base between your thumb and index finger and gently slide down, stretching and twisting as you go and pulling off at the tip. Move along the hand, working each finger and the thumb.

Move to the other hand and repeat steps 1–4.

Neck and Upper Back

This is an easy routine that you can do sitting at a kitchen table, desk or any other stable surface at a suitable height. As the giver, you should be able to work with your arms straight and in the postures shown on pages 22–3. Make you partner comfortable, with their arms and upper body cushioned – a pile of towels or a pillow is ideal.

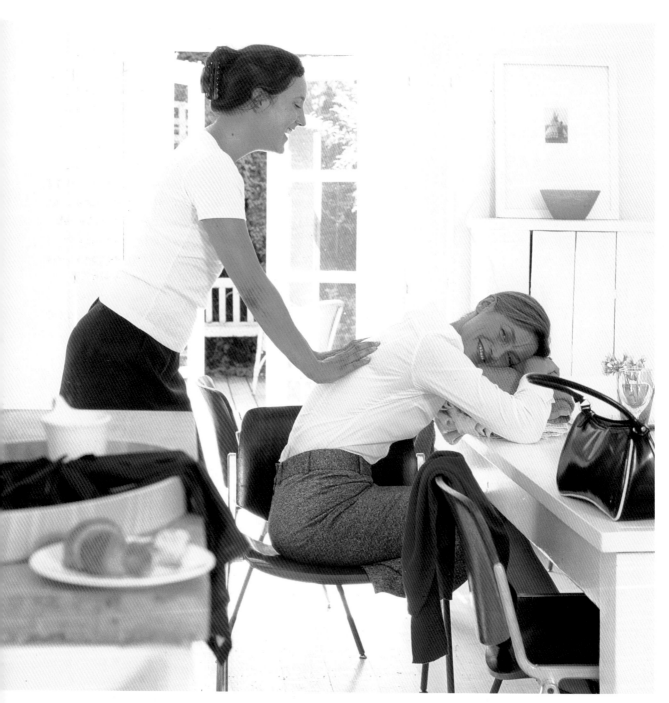

1

Begin by resting your right hand on your partner's right shoulder to make contact. Then, using your left hand, work from the left of the spine outwards, applying steady pressure from the heel of the hand and slowly moving from the lower back up to the top of the shoulder blade.

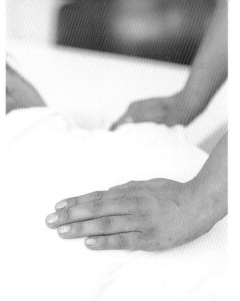

2

Make a fist with the working hand and effleurage (see page 28) in large circles, always applying the pressure on the upward strokes towards the heart.

3

Move side-on to your partner, bring them upright and move your right hand from the right shoulder across to the upper left arm, giving support across the front of the upper torso. With your left hand, lift and squeeze the muscle between the left shoulder blade and the spine with the heel of your hand and fingers.

Move to the other side and repeat steps 1–3.

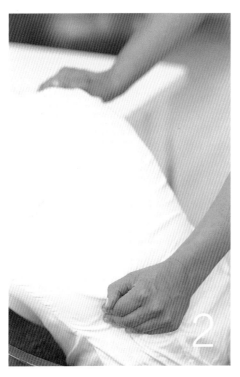

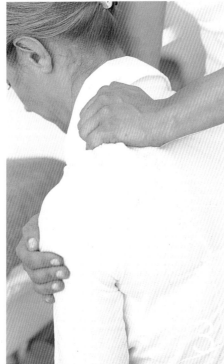

SAFETY FIRST

Remember: always work on either side of the spine, never directly over it.

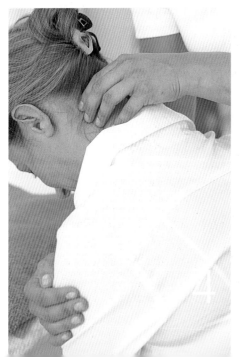

4

Ask your partner to drop their head slightly and, still supporting the front of the shoulders, squeeze the muscles of the neck between your fingers and thumb, working up towards the base of the skull. If you are finishing the massage here, 'ground' your partner by gently squeezing down the arms and legs, and hold the feet for ten seconds.

Upper Arms and Shoulders

After a long day at work tension appears in the muscles which stabilize the shoulder, enabling the arms and hands to work.

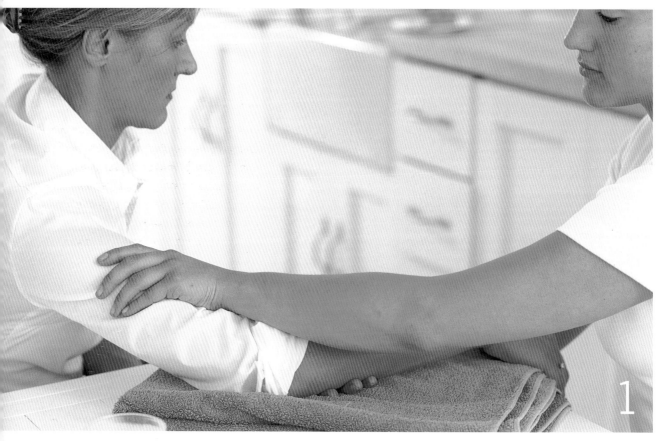

1

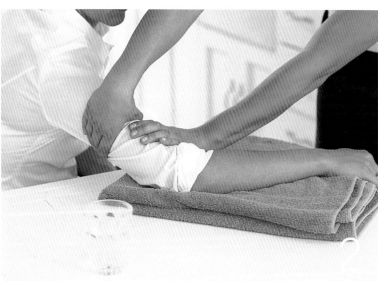

1

With one hand under your partner's elbow for support, effleurage (see page 28) the upper arm from elbow to shoulder, turning your hand at the top and returning down the outside of the arm.

2

Turning side on to your partner, apply the wringing stroke (see page 31) to the muscles of the upper arm, using continuous, rhythmic strokes and covering the whole of the area.

3

Glide upwards from the wrist to the shoulder, applying pressure with your thumb pads and tracing the natural contours of the muscle and skeleton as you go. Repeat three to five times.

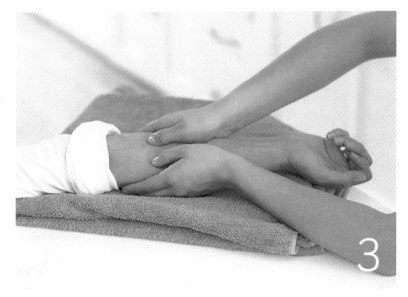

4

With one hand supporting the upper arm and the other holding your partner's hand in a firm grasp, lean back and give a comfortable stretch to your partner's arm and shoulder. Hold for five to ten seconds and then release slowly.

Move to the other arm and repeat steps 1–4.

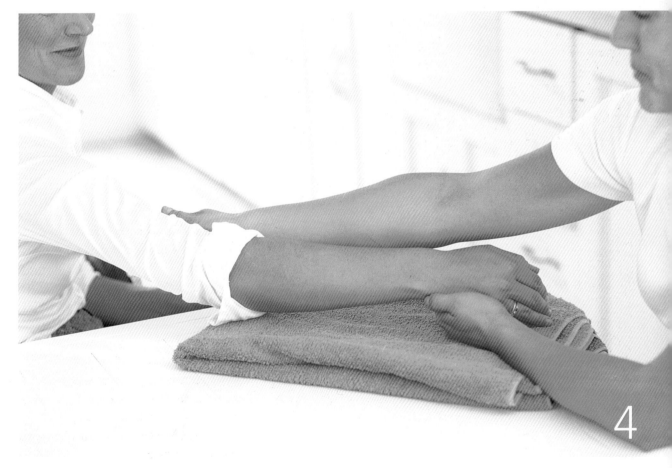

Back

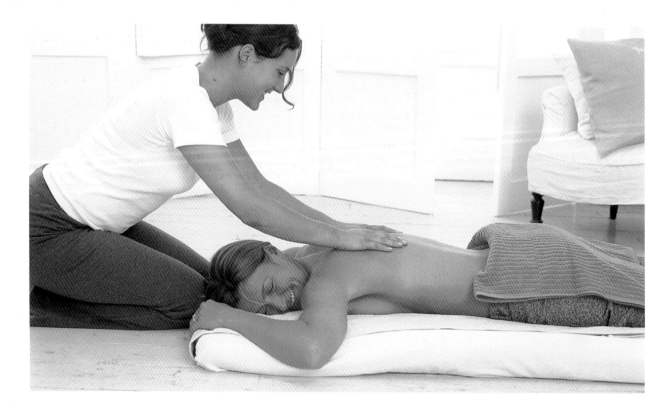

Back pain accounts for more lost working days than any other complaint. The back is vulnerable because it is our main supportive structure and it stores enormous amounts of tension in the large muscles that cover the area. The majority of people visiting a massage therapist will have backache of some kind, usually due to poor posture habits.

The back is the largest single area you will be massaging, and it is often the best place to start a routine, as it enables your partner to relax and not feel the need to engage in conversation. Make sure that you are comfortable and reserve your energy by moving your whole body from the hips rather than just your arms and upper body. You can add the back routine to others that treat the head or legs and buttocks, but it is just as effective on its own.

Once you have made sure that the environment is conducive to massage, position yourself at your partner's head with their arms placed out to the side. With warm hands and warmed oil, place your hands gently on each shoulder blade and hold for ten to twenty seconds in order to put your partner at ease. At this stage you may observe some tightness and rigidity or even the muscles twitching as they start to relax.

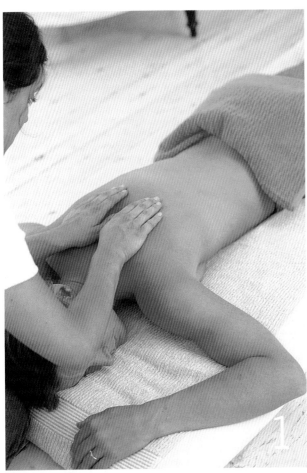

1

Using the flat-handed effleurage stroke (see page 28), work on either side of the spine, gliding your hands downwards to the lower back. If you are working on the floor, you may find it necessary to rise up on your knees in order to drop your weight behind the stroke as you stretch forwards towards the lower back area.

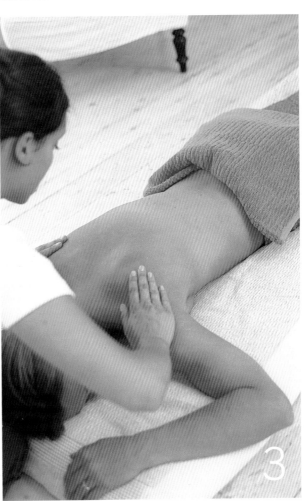

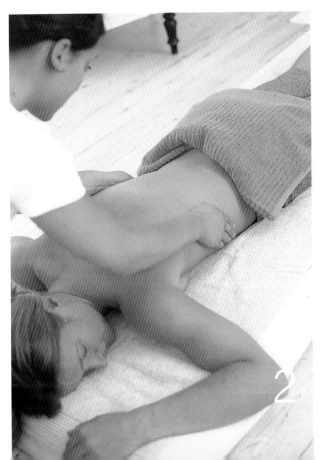

2

At the lower back, glide your hands outwards in opposite directions to the sides of the torso and then bring them up the sides with a slight pull, ending level with the armpit.

3

Bring your hands inwards towards the spine, gliding over the tops of the shoulder blades.

At this stage you can either repeat steps 1–3 four or five times or continue with the sequence.

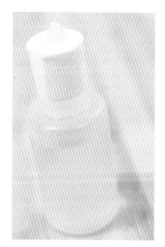

Tip

Transfer your massage oil into a handy spout-topped bottle. This will make it easier to oil your hands before, and during, a massage and avoid any spillage.

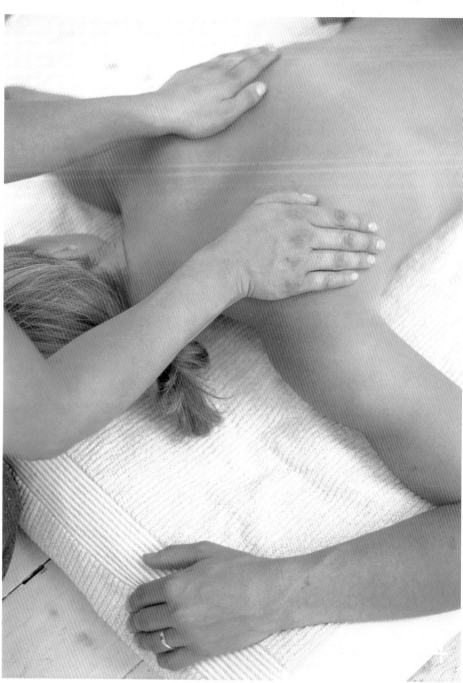

4 & 5

At the shoulder blades turn your hands outwards and bring them over the top of the shoulders, so that the flat of your hands are now turned upwards with the fingers resting on the front of the shoulders. Scoop your hands inwards towards the neck.

Repeat steps 1–4 three or four times. On the final stroke, you may wish to bring your hands up the neck, finishing at the hairline.

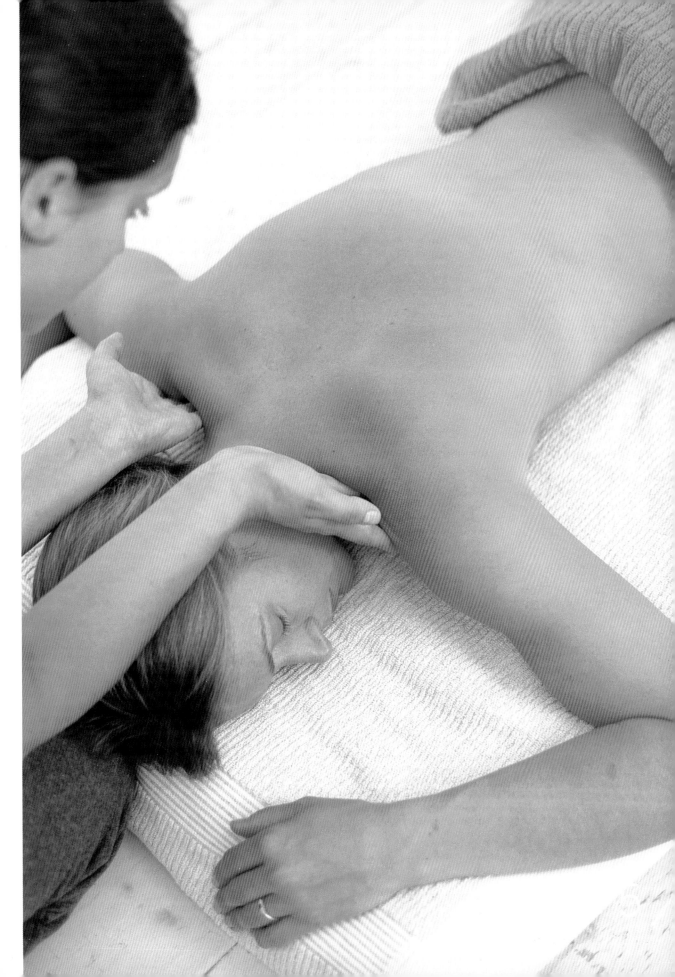

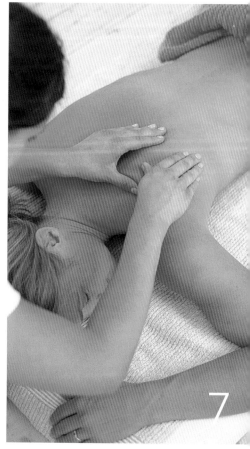

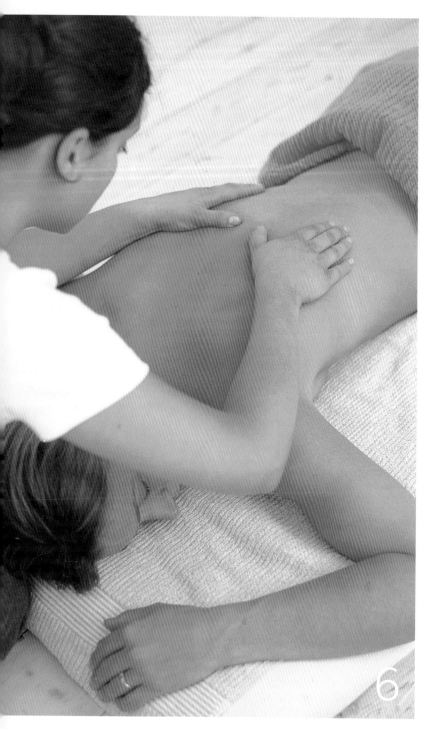

Reverse Effleurage

This routine is called 'reverse effleurage', as you are working in the opposite direction to before. It is a potentially deeper treatment and concentrates on the upper back and shoulder area where tension, discomfort and even pain are often experienced. To work more deeply and break down tension in the area, a variety of strokes can be used following step 3 (see page 105). These are effective in stretching tight muscles and breaking down knots of tension, at the same time promoting relaxation and circulation in the area.

6

Place the flats of your thumbs on either side of the spine and, applying the effleurage stroke, glide each thumb simultaneously downwards to the lower back. You may feel nodules and observe a change of skin tone in particularly tense areas. Repeat three or four times.

7

In the triangle between the spine, the edge of the shoulder blade and the base of the neck, and working on one side and then the other, apply the thumb rolling stroke (see page 35), making sure that you use the entire length of your thumbs and not just the pads. Where you come across knots of tension, spend a little time working on the area and then soothe with lighter, broader strokes.

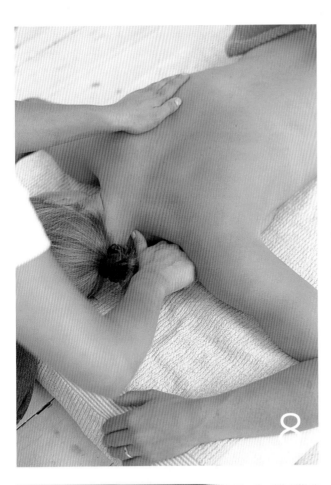

8

For this move, make sure that your partner's head is facing away from the side being massaged. Rest one hand on the upper back and with the other make a fist with your fingers. Using only the flat part of the fist, not the knuckles, glide outwards from the base of the neck to the edge of the shoulder, keeping it flat to the surface. Ease off the pressure at the end of the stroke, lift the hand and return to the base of the neck. Repeat three or four times before moving to the other side. Always adjust the pressure in response to the tightness of the muscle. This is called 'du poing' effleurage and is used for tight or highly developed muscles.

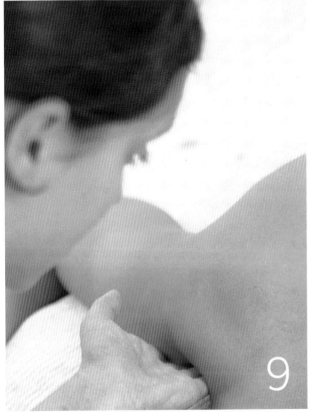

9

Hold and support your partner's head, which should be turned away from the side being massaged. With the web of your hand, glide down the neck with the palm and fingers on the underside, applying gentle pressure and pushing outwards, ending at the top of the arm. Repeat a few times before moving to the other side. If you feel confident, at the same time try moving your partner's head slightly to the opposite side, which applies a very gentle stretch to the muscle fibres and helps to release tension. Do not use the extra stretch if your partner suffers from osteoporosis or spondylosis (inflammation of the vertabrae).

Neck and Shoulders

You can use this routine on its own, or it can be a natural progression from the back massage on pages 104–9. Position your partner on their back and make sure they are comfortable. Place a rolled-up towel under their knees for support and position yourself at their head. It is said that we suppress anger and sorrow by tightening the throat and shoulder muscles, so it is important to devote special care and attention to both the back and the front of these areas.

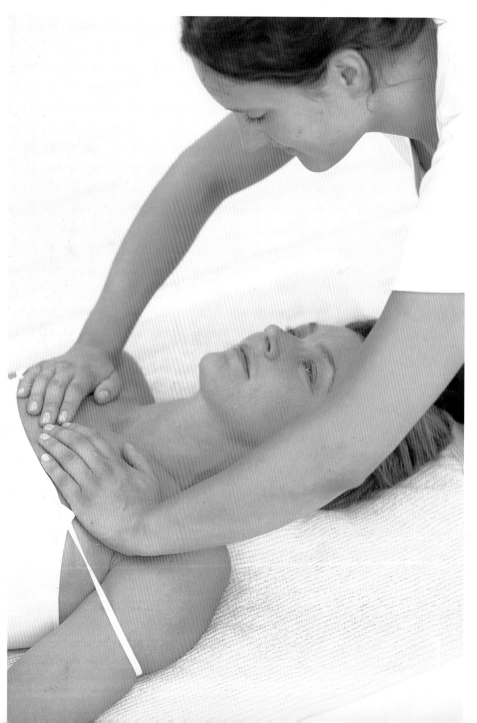

1

Apply oil to your hands and place them gently on the upper chest, just below the collarbone, with your fingers pointing towards each other. Hold this contact for ten seconds and then effleurage (see page 28) by gliding your hands away from each other towards the shoulders in long, sweeping strokes. Do not lean into the chest and apply pressure only on the outward stroke.

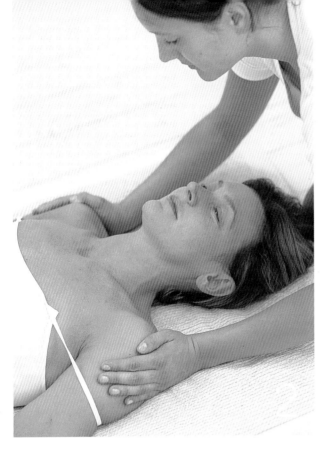

2

On reaching the shoulders, increase the pressure and push them downwards, scooping your hands underneath ready for the return stroke. This gives the neck and shoulders a good frontal stretch.

3

With your hands now palm up, continue the stroke, bringing them up underneath the neck until they overlap.

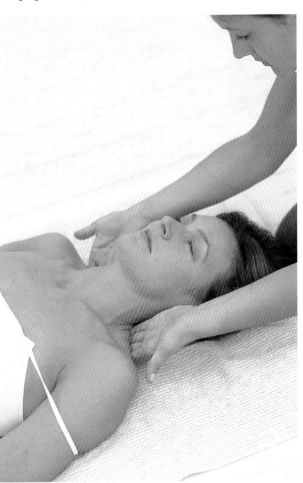

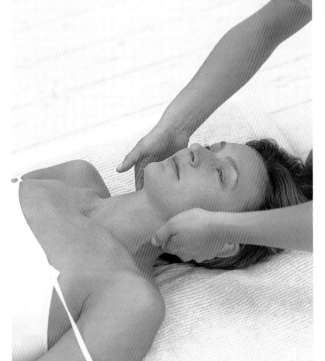

4

Cup your hands under the neck, close to the base of the skull. Pull them towards you slowly, at the same time leaning back slightly to facilitate a very gentle neck stretch without lifting the head. Release slowly.

Repeat steps 1–4 three or four times, and on the last stroke continue from the neck up the back of the head and off.

5

Now use the 'du poing' effleurage stroke (see step 8 on page 109). Ensure that your partner's head is not facing the side being worked on, then rest one hand on their shoulder and with the other glide outwards with the flat of your fist along the back of the shoulder from the base of the neck to the top of the arm, keeping it flat to the surface. Ease off the pressure at the end of the stroke, lift your hand and return to the base of the neck. Repeat three or four times.

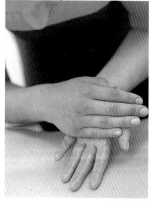

Tip

Hand cream or massage oil applied to the palms of your own hands will make the experience more pleasant for your partner. Don't forget to warm your hands before making contact.

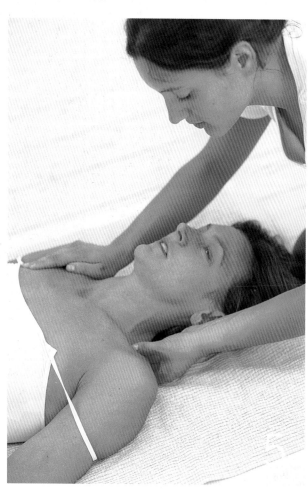

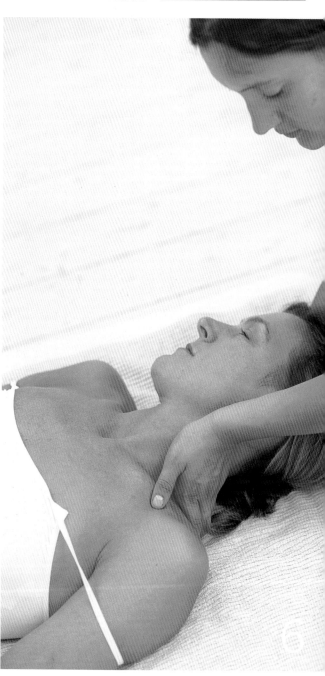

6

Following step 9 on page 109, hold and support your partner's head, which should be turned away from the side being massaged. With the web of your hand, glide down the neck with the palm and fingers on the underside, applying gentle pressure and pushing outwards, ending at the top of the arm. Repeat three or four times. Move to the other side and repeat steps 5 and 6.

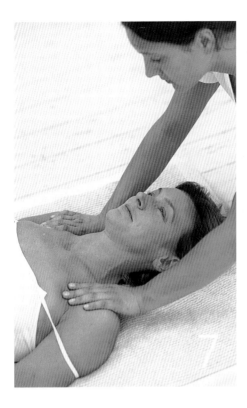

7

Place your hands on your partner's shoulders and, using a firm pressure, alternately push down and then release in a continuous movement, one hand pushing while the other releases. Repeat several times.

8

Move your hands up either side of the neck until the pads of your fingers rest on the ridge at the base of the skull. Lean back gently and with the pads of your fingers apply pressure in a circular motion, at the same time rotating your fingers. On the final stroke, comb your fingers through your partner's hair to the top of the head and pull off.

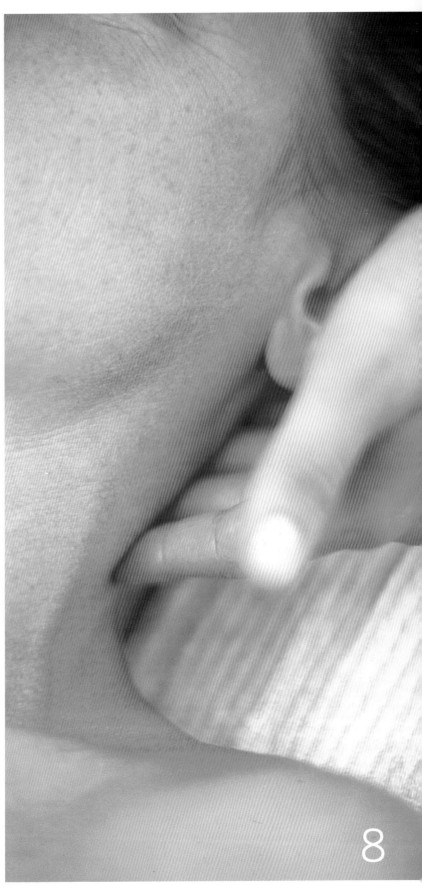

Eyes

In today's world of computer screens, electronic media and bright lights, eye strain can cause blurred vision, headaches and even migraines. To counteract this, there is a simple routine that you can do after work or even during the day while sitting at a table or desk. Make sure you are sitting comfortably with your elbows on a firm surface so that you can hold the weight of your head in your hands. Oil is not necessary, although a small amount of rose absolute would add a special dimension to the massage.

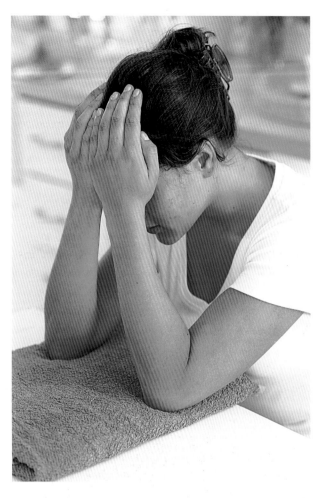

1

Place your fingers on the top of your head, rest your eyes into the heels of your hands and relax your whole body, letting your hands take the weight. Hold this position for 20 seconds and release. Repeat four times.

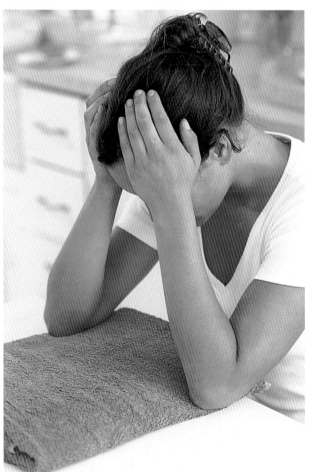

2

Move the heels of your hands to rest on your eyebrows. Take a deep breath, and on the out breath glide your hands from the inner ends of your eyebrows outwards and pull off at the side of the head, smoothing the entire browline. Repeat four times.

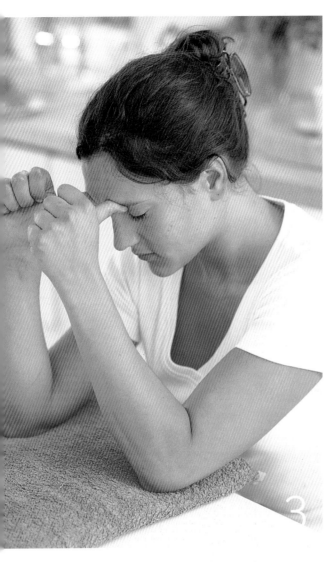

3

Move back to the inner ends of the eyebrows and place the pads of your thumbs underneath the inner edge. As this is a very tender area, do not lean in with the whole weight of your head but stick to a level of pressure with which you are comfortable. Hold for ten seconds and release. Repeat four times. This technique is not only good for tired eyes but also helps to clear congestion of the sinuses and related headaches.

4

Finally, place the middle two fingers of each hand on your temples and, using the pressure from your fingers as support, release your head and neck. Take a deep breath, and on the out breath very slowly rotate your fingers clockwise. Repeat the movement four times. You can also apply the pressure directly to your temples without rotating your fingers.

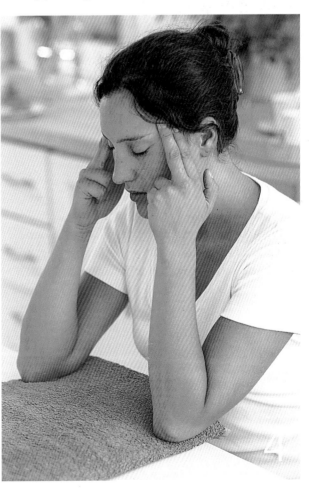

Tip

If you spend the working day sitting in front of a computer screen, relieve the strain on your eyes by carrying out a few simple techniques when you get home in the evening.

Self-massage

One of the best ways of combating stress and repetitive strain injury (see page 98) is to take regular breaks during your working day. Here is a simple routine that can be done while you are at work – all you need is a stable surface, such as a desk, and a little time. Repeat each movement as many times as you feel necessary in the time you have available – whether you spend five minutes or twenty minutes working on yourself, you will definitely feel the benefit and have more energy for the rest of the day. This routine is particularly good for neck tension, which often causes headaches or a feeling of stiffness.

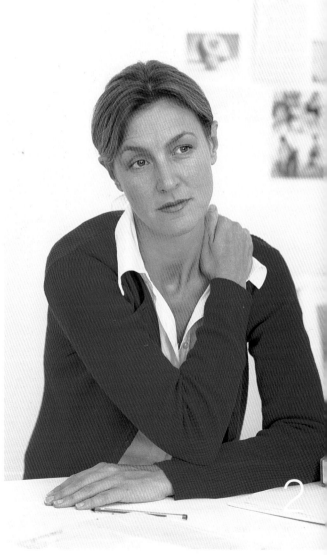

1

Resting your elbows on the desk, place your fingers at the back of your neck behind your ears, leaning your head forward slightly. Make sure you are comfortable, and then with the pads of your fingers work the length of your neck on either side of the vertebrae by rotating your fingers and applying pressure at the same time.

2

Place one hand on the desk and the other on the opposite shoulder. Tilting your head slightly away from the area you are massaging, squeeze the muscle between the fingers and heel of your hand, working from the base of the neck to the edge of the shoulder.

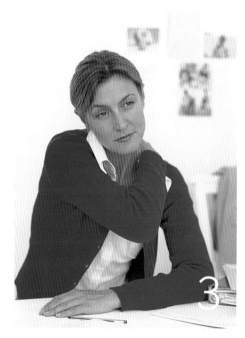

3

In the same position as for step 2, place your fingers on the top of the shoulder muscle and rotate the pads of your fingers while applying pressure, again working from the base of the neck to the edge of the shoulder.

Move to the other side and repeat steps 2 and 3.

4

To complete the massage, take the lobe of your ears between your thumb and index finger, close your eyes and visualize a calming scene – a walk along a beach, perhaps, or sitting in a garden. Take a deep breath, and on the out breath pull downwards and off very slowly. Have a drink of water and you will now feel ready to continue your work.

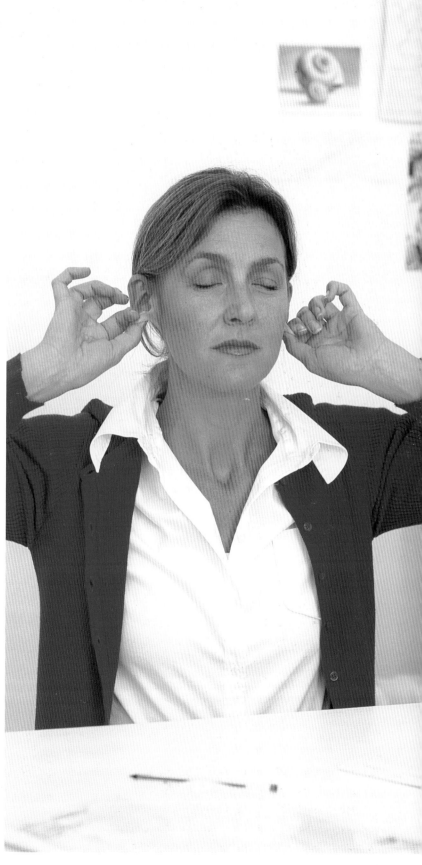

Seated routine

If you have a reasonable amount of time to spare – during your lunch break, for instance – this seated routine through the clothes will allow you to work on the back as well as the neck and shoulders, which are the main areas of tension suffered by office and computer workers. These days, large organizations often employ a 'corporate' or 'on-site' massage therapist as part of their health programme, and a specially designed chair is used for the comfort of the receiver and accessibility for the giver. This seated routine adapts an ordinary office chair for the purpose, but take care to use one without wheels!

1

Start by making your partner feel comfortable with your touch. Bring both hands down slowly and place them palm down on your partner's shoulders. Hold for 30 seconds, while your partner closes their eyes and relaxes in preparation for the massage.

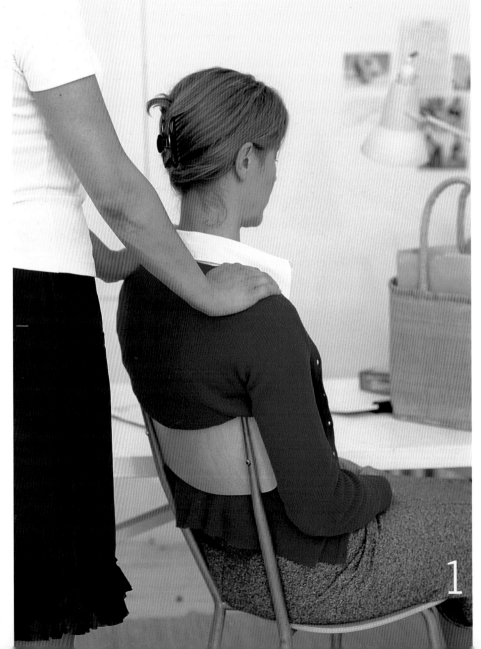

1

2

Working the whole area between the spine and the shoulder blades, use the heel of your hands and your fingers to lift and squeeze the muscle at the same time. Repeat this (and the following steps) three to five times.

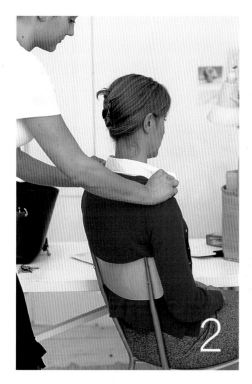

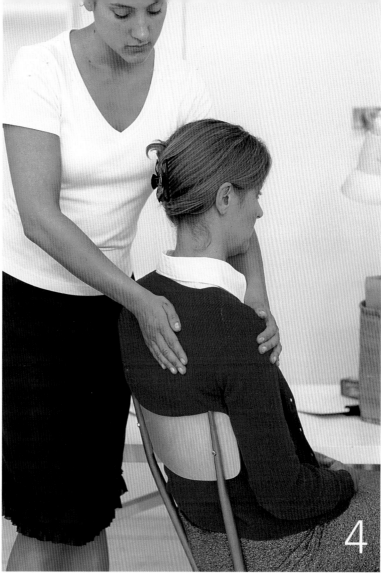

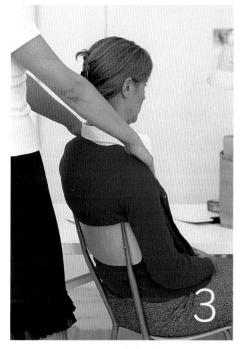

3

Placing your fingers over the shoulders, rotate the pads of your fingers across the muscle in the triangle between the collarbone and shoulder. Lean back slightly as you do this stroke to apply pressure – the further you lean back, the stronger the pull, but always stick to a level that is comfortable for your partner.

4

Move so that you are side-on to your partner and place one arm across their upper chest area for support. Use the heel of your other hand to massage in circular movements over the back and shoulder area. It is a good idea to vary the speed from a gentle to a quite invigorating pace. This will really warm up the muscles and increase the flow of both blood and lymph.

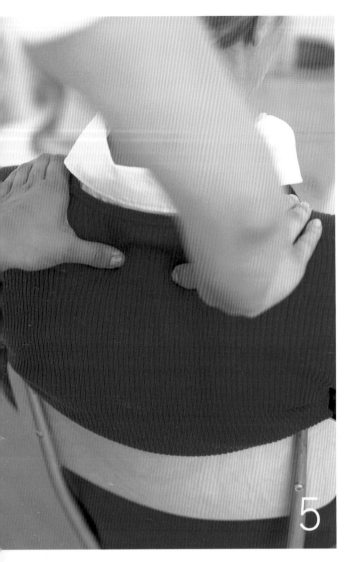

5

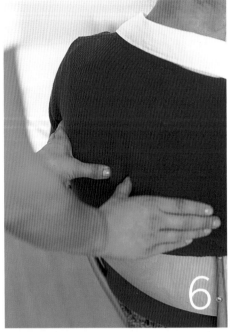

6

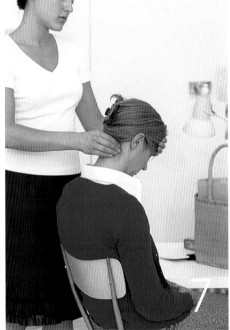

7

5

Now that the muscles are more relaxed, kneading and deeper pressure can be applied. Stand straight on to your partner and, with your thumbs placed on either side of the spine and using the pads only, apply on-the-spot pressure at 3cm (1¼in) intervals along the tops of the shoulder muscles, working outwards and then returning.

6

Using the same technique as in step 5, press your thumbs simultaneously on either side of the spine, working slowly down to the lower back area and then returning. If you want to reach lower, where most people experience discomfort, you can get your partner to straddle the chair (see page 82).

7

Move to the side of your partner and support their forehead with the hand nearest to them. Ask them to rest their head on your hand and then place your free hand on the back of the neck area and squeeze the muscles between your fingers and thumb. Work upwards to the base of the skull, then slide your fingers back to the starting position, ready to repeat.

8

Return to your position behind your partner and, standing straight, place the backs of your forearms on the top of the shoulders so that your palms are facing upwards. Make sure your wrists are relaxed, take a deep breath, and on the out breath lean gently and slowly into the muscle, hold and then release. Work with your breathing – keep the pressure on for the duration of your out breath and release it with your in breath.

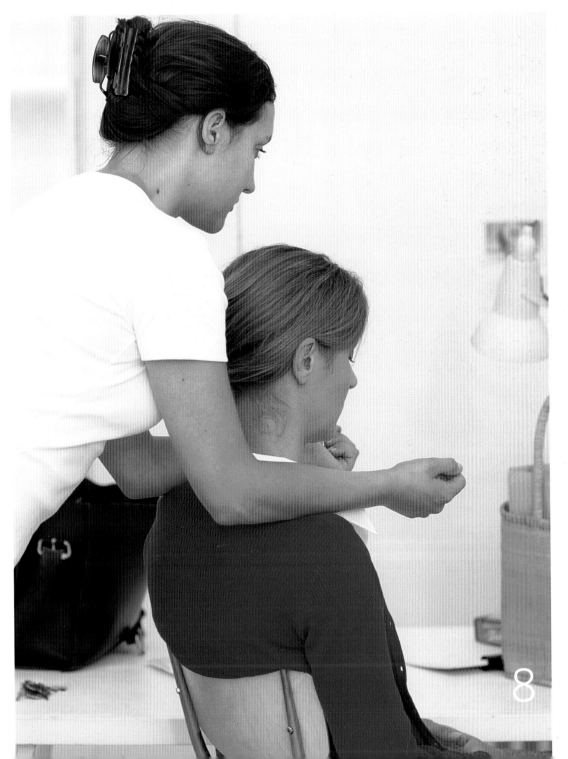

8

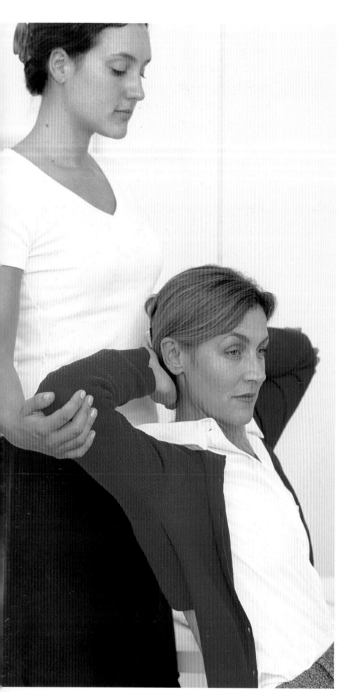

10

Starting to bring the routine to a close, rest your hands lightly on the crown of your partner's head and stroke with a hand-over-hand motion from the forehead over to the base of the neck and down the back.

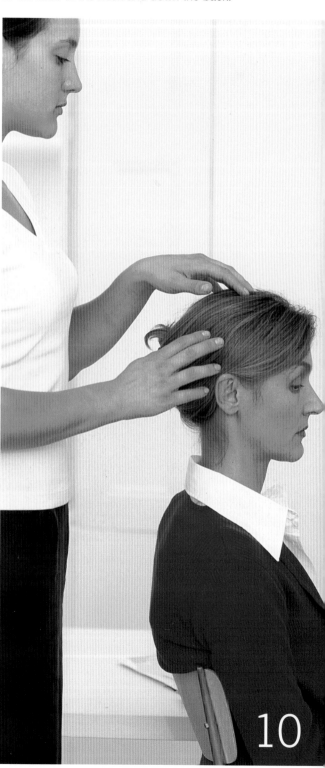

10

9

Remaining in the same position, ask your partner to clasp their hands behind their head, level with their ears. Hold each elbow firmly with your hands and ask your partner to take a deep breath. As they breath out, slowly pull their arms straight back towards you to a comfortable point of resistance, hold for five seconds and then release. This will give an excellent stretch to the front chest and open up the respiratory area.

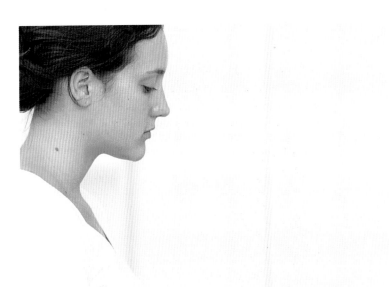

12

Finish off with a 'grounding' movement (see page 39) by holding your partner's feet with thumb pressure on the instep. This will bring them 'back to earth', otherwise they may feel a little light-headed and 'spacey'. Remember to offer them a drink of water when you have finished and before they return to their desk.

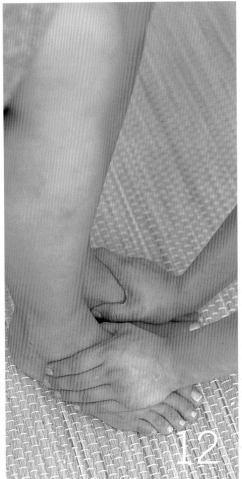

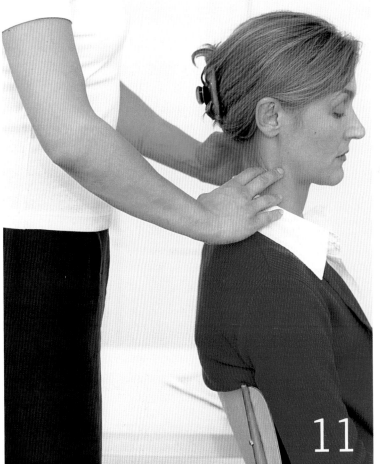

11

With both hands working simultaneously, move down the sides of the head and tops of the shoulders in a gentle stroking movement, then squeeze down the arms to the elbow.

Stress Management

Most of us feel stressed at some times in our lives whether we are physically exhausted or mentally overwrought, the key is how we manage and overcome those feelings. When we are relaxed we can deal with most of the day-to-day lows and highs, whereas when we are under stress, a simple hurdle can become a mountain.

SOME MENTAL SIGNS OF STRESS

- Being unfocused
- Forgetfulness
- Indecisiveness
- Being disorganized
- Loss of short-term memory
- Making errors
- Misjudgments
- Finding simple tasks difficult
- Experiencing mood swings
- Tearfulness
- Negativity
- Excessive worrying
- Panic attacks

SOME PHYSICAL SIGNS OF STRESS

- Tension
- Headaches and migraines
- Shallow breathing
- Palpitations
- Dry mouth
- Sweating
- Nausea
- Sleeping problems
- Restlessness
- Shakiness or dizziness
- Indigestion
- Ulcers
- Back and neck ache

How Do We Get Stressed?

Sustained work overload at home or work is a common cause, but other events, such as financial difficulties, problems with the family, serious illness or the breakdown of a relationship – anything that changes your daily routine drastically – could induce stress.

Stress Levels

Most experts say that a small amount of stress is necessary and beneficial. It motivates and stimulates our lives, and we need to be able to address daily situations to make us stronger to deal with larger changes. Sometimes, however, stresses become too great or erode the spirit over a period, and this can even bring on illness and, in the extreme, a physical or emotional breakdown.

Who Does Stress Affect?

Some personality types are more susceptible to stress than others and different types of people react to crises in different ways. The 'anxious' person may have a lower stress level than the 'ambitious' person, while some, like the 'perfectionist', create their own, sometimes unnecessary, stress. No matter what type of person you are, the physical reactions are the same, not just in the mind but in blood chemistry, and although they are activated by the sympathetic nervous system, your mind will determine the strength of your physical reaction. The parasympathetic nervous system has the task of helping the body to recover and reversing the physical reactions.

How to Manage Stress

BREATHING:
If you are suffering from stress, correct breathing will enable your body to regain its natural balance, will reduce anxiety and will help you relax. Breathe in deeply, right down to the belly area and then fill the chest cavity. On the out breath push the air out of your mouth from the top of the lungs first and then the belly. Practise this technique, taking long, slow, coordinated inhalations and exhalations and notice how your tense shoulders will drop on the out breath.

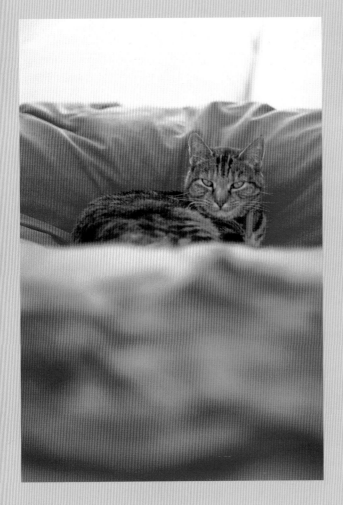

REST:
Each time you finish a work project give yourself a short break. If you can take a short walk or stretch, change the area you are in, have a snack or even close your eyes for a few seconds to clear your mind.

RELAX THE MIND:
It is harder to relax the mind than to rest the body, and you may need to practise the art of visualization. Close your eyes and picture something you find relaxing, such as a holiday you really enjoyed, childhood feelings of no responsibilities or a pretty country cottage away from all the hustle and bustle.

SLEEP:
Sleeping is a great way to relax the mind but is hard to achieve when your mind is racing with worries. Make your bedroom your retreat, do not discuss issues of the day and try to establish a routine. A warm bath and a herbal tea before bed do wonders, then listen to the radio or a talking book so that you can lie with your eyes closed and drift off. Do whatever works best for you.

BE POSITIVE:
It is easy to say 'be positive', and you may wake up feeling positive. Within a few hours, however, you are drained of that energy by the stressful events taking place. First, you must feel good about yourself; we are often very bad at this, so spend time thinking about what you have achieved and not what you haven't done. Second, don't use negative words and always speak about what you are doing or feeling now. Tell yourself you are calm and focused, you are doing your best and you are having a good day, and be amazed by how much you will open yourself to positive change.

LIFESTYLE CHANGES:
When we are under stress we do all the wrong things that ultimately increase our stress – eating badly, not exercising, drinking too much, having no playtime and no structure, for example. Eat sensibly with fewer carbohydrates and more antioxidants and magnesium; drink lots of water (at least six to eight glasses a day) to rehydrate our bodies that are 75 per cent water; reduce your intake of caffeine and alcohol; take up some kind of exercise (even ten minutes every other day will achieve good results); make time to have a social life away from the areas that are causing you stress and when you do have to work have a plan and make a rule that you will complete one task at a time so that at least every work day you will have achieved something.

MASSAGE:
Last but not least, regular massage will give you time and space totally for yourself. It will help reduce physical tension and naturally raise your endorphin levels, making you feel more positive and even euphoric.

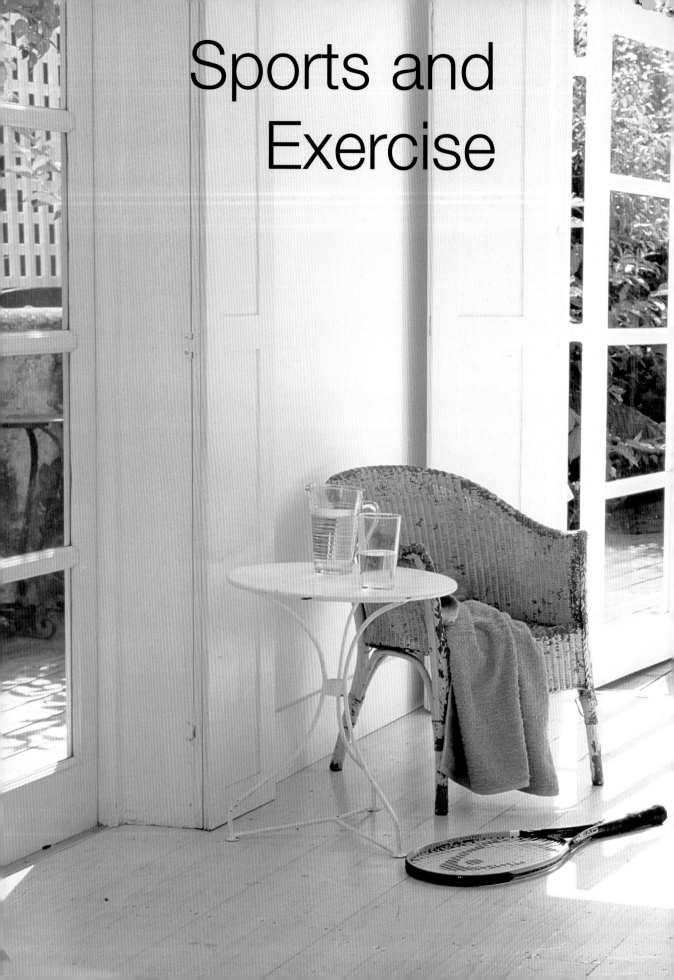

Sports and Exercise

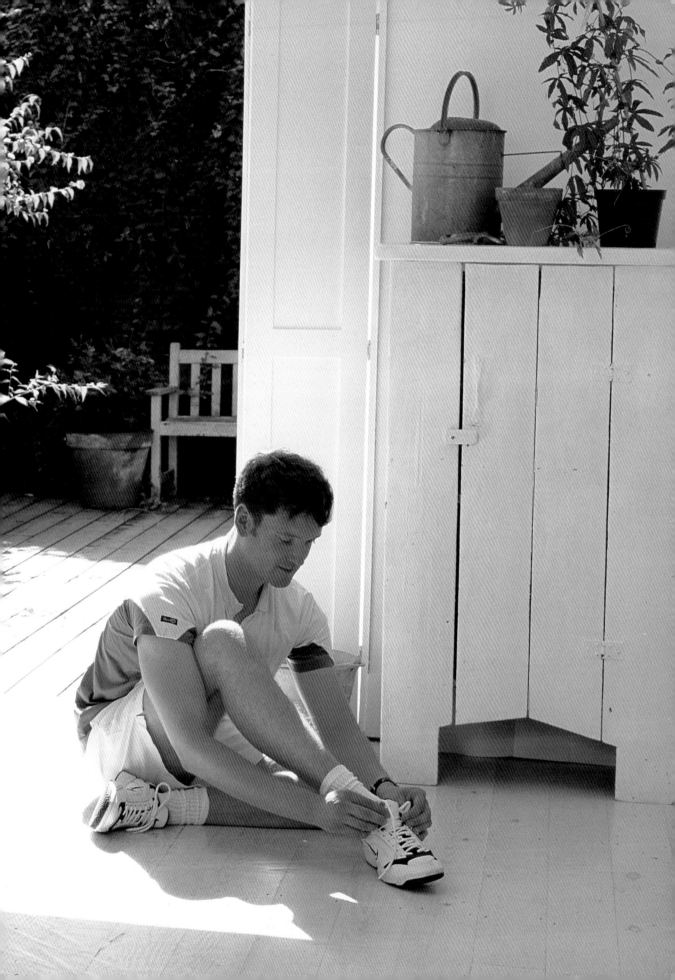

Pre-event Routine

For sports and exercise at all levels, massage can play a beneficial role in preparing the body by helping to condition and tone the muscles. By addressing pockets of tension, problems such as cramp and stiffness can also be prevented. Professional athletes claim that massage can increase the efficiency of their performance by up to 20 per cent, and trained sports massage therapists combine old knowledge with new scientific understanding to provide that extra ingredient.

Massage should preferably be carried out the day before playing sport or exercising, warming up the muscles with effleurage and friction strokes (see pages 28 and 34). Petrissage (see page 30) can also be used but with light pressure only. Passive stretching (see page 36) is also good but should supplement, rather than replace, a warm-up routine.

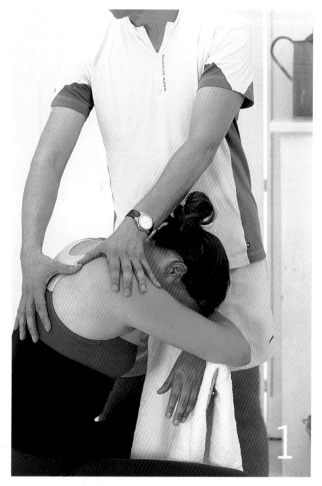

1

1

With your partner sitting astride a chair (see page 13), stand in front and to one side of them so that you can comfortably reach over to the opposite shoulder. Standing straight, with your feet slightly apart, place your thumbs together between the spine and the edge of the shoulder blade and lean into the area, keeping your hands and wrists straight so that your body weight is directed to your thumb pads. Slide your thumbs over the shoulder blade in an effleurage stroke. Repeat three to five times.

Shoulders

You can pay special attention to the muscles that will be used the most. The routine provided here shows you how to work more deeply on the shoulder area, which is most often affected by movements using the upper body, as in racket sports, cricket and golf. These movements will stretch muscle fibres, help to break down nodules and encourage the muscles to relax.

2

Move to the side you are working on and repeat the thumb effleurage over the shoulder blade in the opposite direction, towards the edge of the spine. Repeat three to five times.

3

Rest one hand on the top of the shoulder and place the thumb pad of the other hand between the side of the spine and the top of the shoulder blade. Keeping flat to the surface, glide downwards in 5cm (2in) strokes, gradually adding pressure until the upper back area has been covered. Make sure that you work to a comfortable point so that you do not strain your own back.

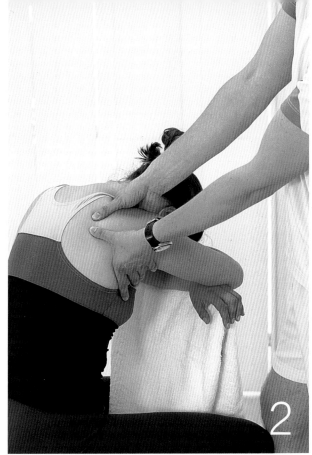

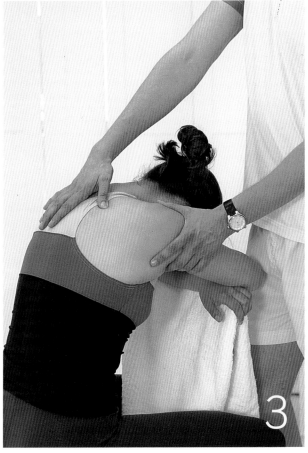

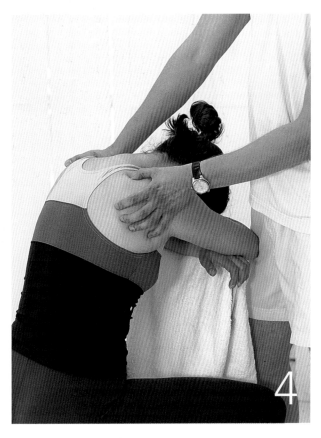

4

Again with one hand resting on the shoulder, apply circular friction to the shoulder blade area with your fingers slightly apart, moving the finger pads in a circular movement and applying even pressure with each finger.

Move to the other side and repeat steps 1–4.

Back

For general exercise the whole of the back area will feel much more supple if the muscles have been relaxed, improving the range of movement and so making the receiver less susceptible to injury. These moves enable you to cover the whole of the back smoothly and with ease, at the same time applying deep pressure without straining your own wrists and hands.

1

With your partner sitting astride a chair (see page 13), stand behind them in the 'warrior' position (see page 23). With straight arms, place one hand on top of the other in the centre of your partner's back and lean your body weight inwards. Hold for about ten seconds.

SAFETY FIRST

Remember: always work on either side of the spine, never directly over it.

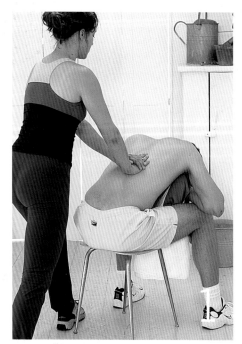

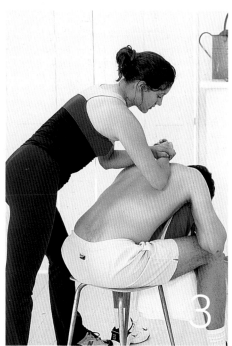

2

Slide one forearm flat to the surface of the back at a right angle to your upper arm, with the opposite hand on top just above the wrist for support. To facilitate this move, bend the knee of the opposite leg forwards towards your working arm.

3

With pressure being applied through your forearm, guided by your holding hand, effleurage (see page 28) in a large, sweeping circle over your partner's back on the side on which you are working. Repeat three to five times.

4

Still holding your upper wrist for support, straighten your arm and pull off slowly.

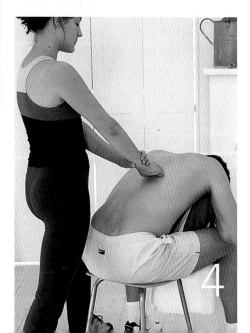

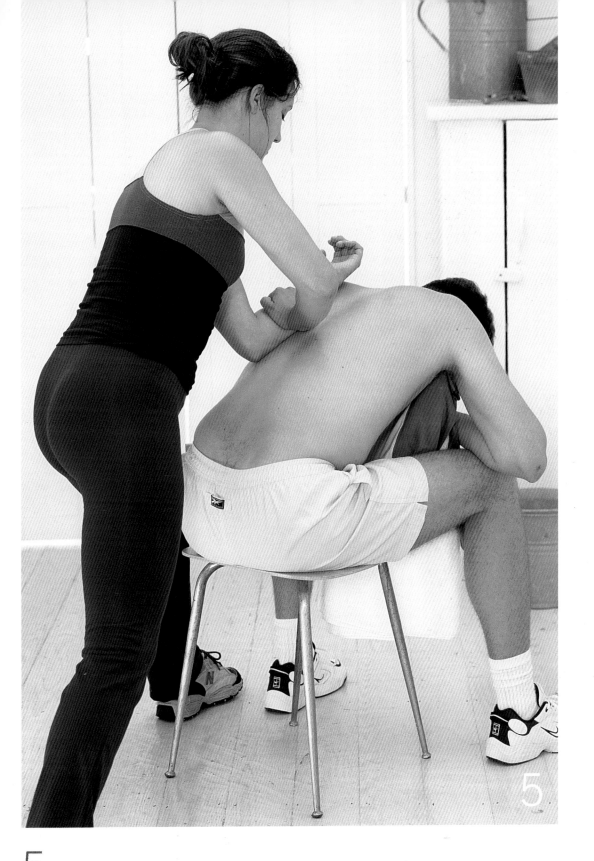

5

Following steps 1–4, change arms and
repeat on the other side of the back.

During Activity

Joint stretching and mobilization techniques are the most effective way of keeping the body conditioned during sports and exercise. These positions were initially devised for dancers, but they can be applied to any activity. You can even integrate them into your warm-up routine.

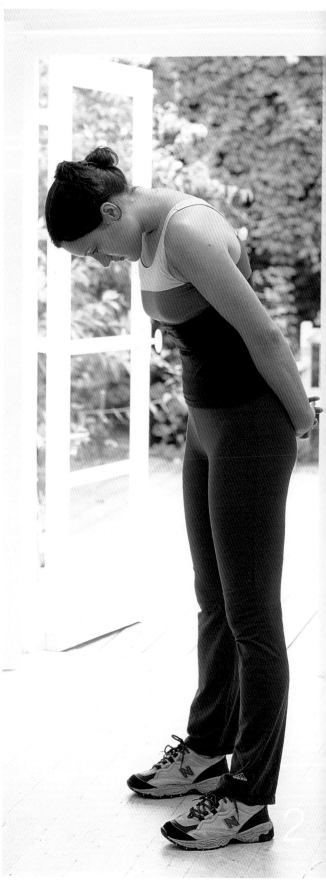

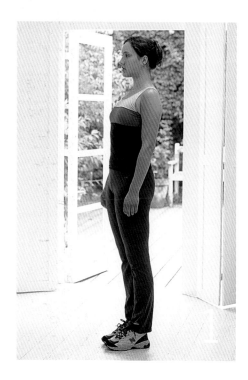

1

Standing straight, shake your arms and hands to relax, then drop them to your sides.

2

Move your feet to the width of your hips and clasp your hands behind your back, tilting your head and upper torso slightly to facilitate this.

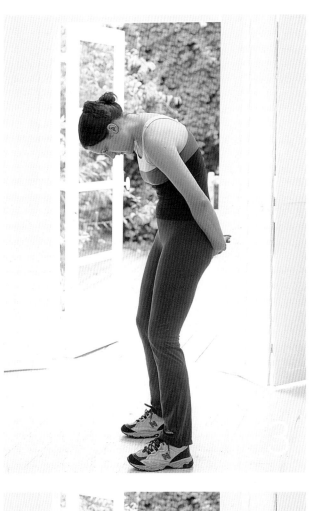

3

Bending your knees, slide your clasped hands lower down, at the same time rounding forward and stretching out your back.

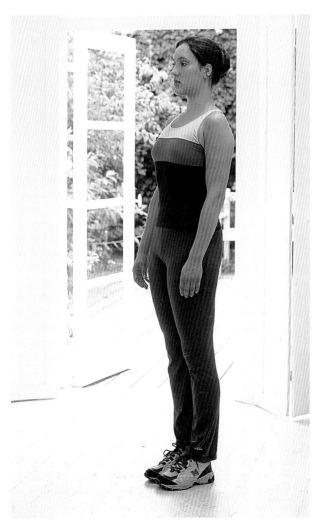

4

Keeping your knees bent, hinge forward and bring your hands around and place them on your thighs just above the knee.

5

Slowly round up and at the same time pull your navel backwards. This will help to lift the spine and return you to your starting position.

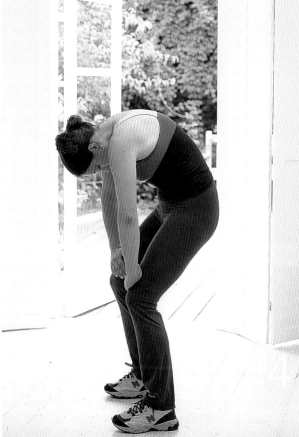

After Exercise

After vigorous exercise waste products, such as lactic acid, will have accumulated in the muscles, and massage can help to disperse these toxins more quickly than simple rest. By bringing fresh blood to tired muscles and replenishing oxygen and nutrients, recovery is much faster. However, it is advisable to wait for 1–1½ hours following exercise before massaging. To soothe tired limbs, use long, light strokes to work over the whole body. Be sensitive to any particularly sore areas and increase pressure gently to disperse the build-up of toxins.

Buttocks

The buttocks house the gluteus muscles, which can often stiffen up after exercise that uses the lower body, such as walking, running, climbing or cycling. Localized massage can reduce the 'tight' feeling and restore muscle function.

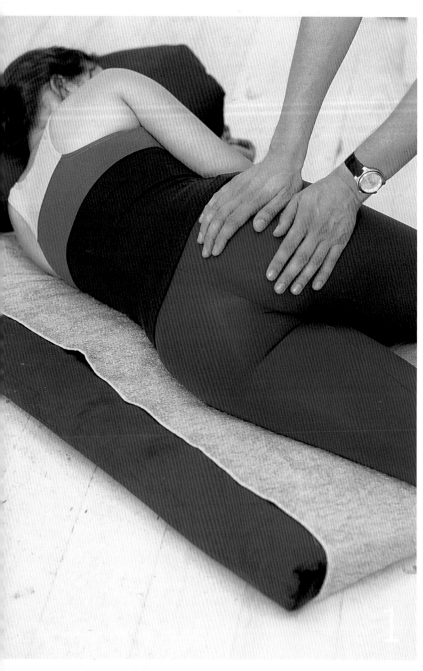

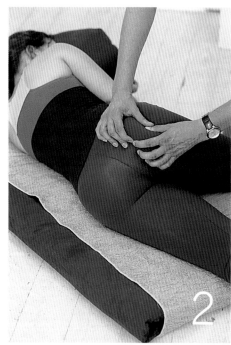

1
Position yourself facing your partner from the side, place the flat of your hands on the buttock area and effleurage (see page 28) the area all over.

2
With both hands, take hold of the muscle between your fingers and thumbs and, lifting and squeezing, work your way across the length of the muscle.

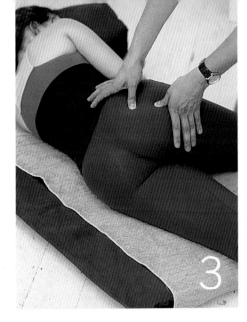

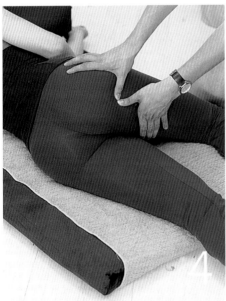

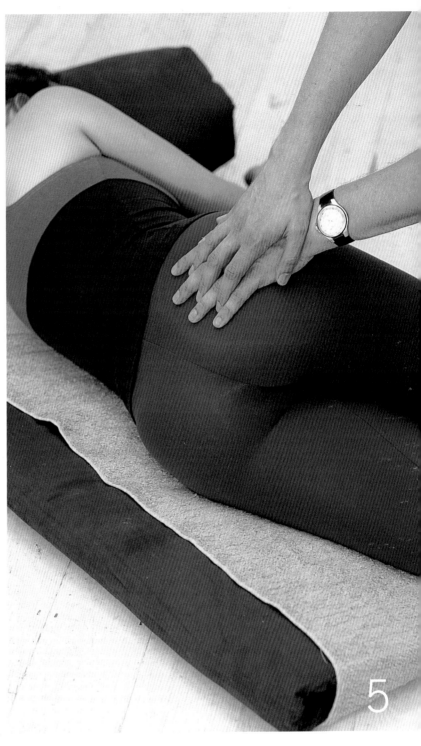

3

Place both thumb pads around the top of the muscle and apply the thumb rolling stroke (see page 35) around the border of the gluteus.

4

Place both thumbs on the pressure point in the centre of the buttock crease, lean your body weight in and hold for three to five seconds. Repeat three times. This movement helps to relax the muscles of the hips and lower back.

5

Finally, place one hand on top of the other and, leaning in, apply the double-handed effleurage stroke (see step 2, page 45) over the whole area, holding for a moment before pulling off.

Move to the other side and repeat steps 1–5.

3

Using the same hand positions as in step 2 and starting from above the knee, glide up the thigh as far as is comfortable and using discretion, returning with a flat-handed stroke down the side of the leg to the knee.

Repeat steps 1–3 three or four times.

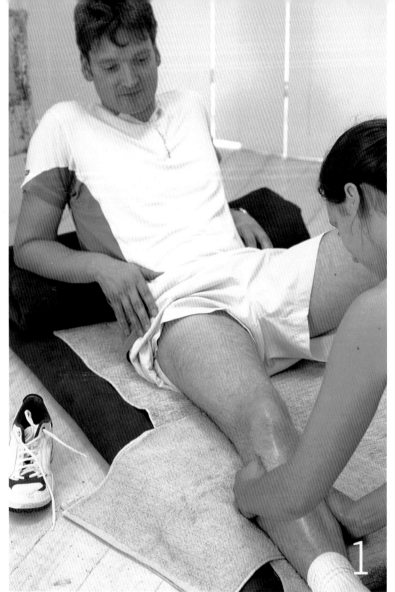

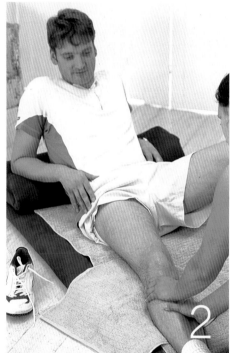

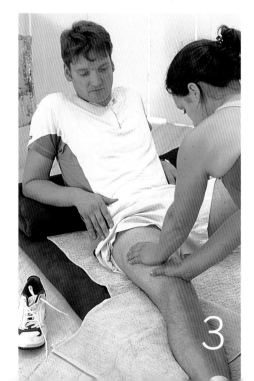

Legs

The legs are very vulnerable during activities such as ball games, skiing and skating.

1

Start with a gentle effleurage stroke (see page 28). Position yourself at the foot of your partner and glide upwards from the ankle to the thigh without overstretching yourself, lifting off the pressure over the knee.

2

Place the web of your hand on the top of the lower leg, with fingers and thumb on the muscle either side, making a V shape. Place your other hand behind the first slightly lower down the leg in the same position, then glide up the leg to just below the knee and return with flat hands down the side of the leg, ready to repeat.

4

With your fingers hooked on either side of the knee joint, apply pressure with your thumbs to the spaces around the knee, working in opposite directions from top to bottom and then return. Repeat, but instead of direct pressure, rotate your thumbs slowly, working around the knee as before.

Move to the other leg and repeat steps 1–4, then finish by 'grounding' your partner (see page 39).

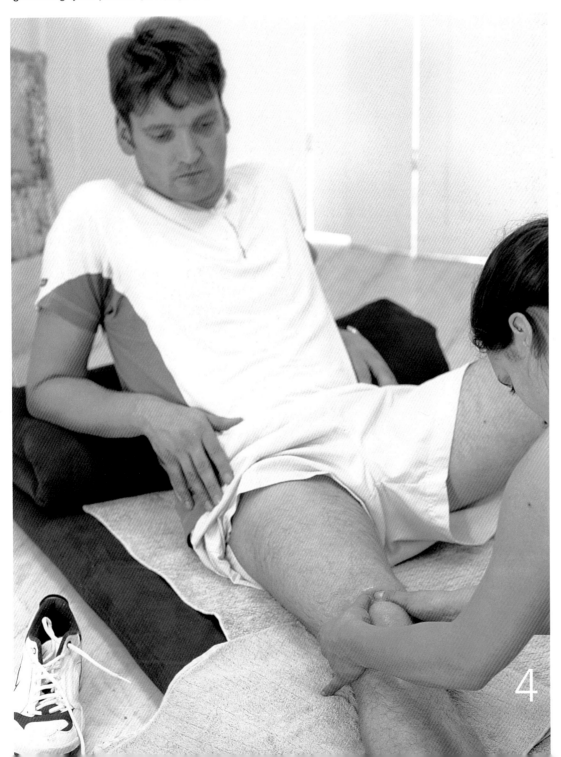

4

Strains

Strains and sprains are common injuries during sport and exercise and involve a tear in the muscle, usually caused by overdoing exercise, over-stretching or a bad movement. Massage helps by reducing the swelling that is a visible symptom of this type of injury – always work above the swelling and if the skin reddens, work higher. Reducing the swelling will automatically reduce pain as well; however, if the area feels too sensitive to receive massage, you could palpate pressure points to achieve the same results (see page 17).

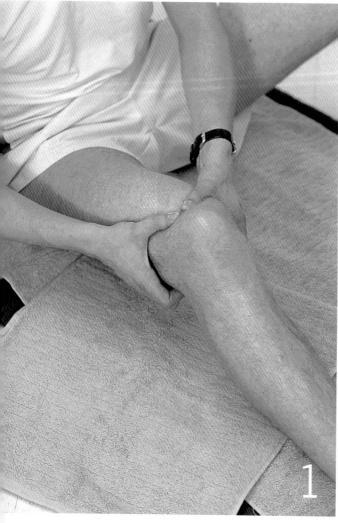

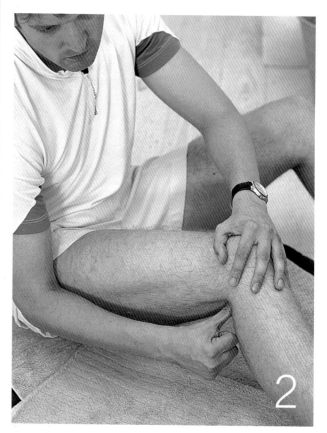

1

Place your hands on either side of your knee with your fingers hooked underneath for support and your thumbs on the top of the leg, just above the knee. Press inwards two or three times, holding the pressure for three to five seconds each time.

2

Holding the top of the knee with one hand for support, bend slightly and place the thumb of your other hand in the hollow above the ridge of the bone in the lower leg (femur) near the crease. As in step 1, press inwards two or three times, holding the pressure for three to five seconds each time.

Aching Pecs

The broad, flat area at the front of the chest on either side of the breast bone houses the pectoral muscles, which connect the ribcage, the collar bone and the top of the bone in the upper arm (humerus). Over-exercising the upper torso puts a strain on these large muscles and causes discomfort. Weight lifting, boxing and body building are sports in which this type of strain is a common occurrence.

1

Working side-on to your partner, place the flat of both your hands on the central chest in line with the lower ribs and, using the effleurage stroke (see page 28), glide your hands sideways up the chest, across the top of the shoulder to the outer edge and down the outer side of the upper torso, back to where you started. Repeat several times.

2

Keeping one hand on the centre chest, place the hand nearest to your partner's head on the pectoral muscle furthest away from you and, using the whole hand but applying firm pressure from the heel, glide the width of the muscle, stroking your fingers over the top of the arm. Return with reduced pressure. Repeat several times.

3

Moving to a position above your partner's head, lean forwards and place your hands on the pectoral muscles, with your fingers pointing to the edge of the chest. With your arms straight, apply firm pressure and stretch each muscle with a slight push downwards. Take care not to slide off, as this is a press-and-stretch move rather than a glide. Repeat several times.

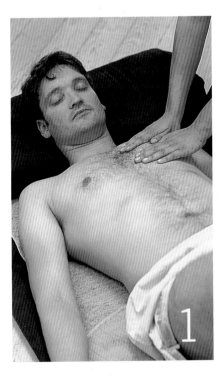

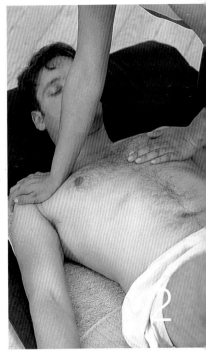

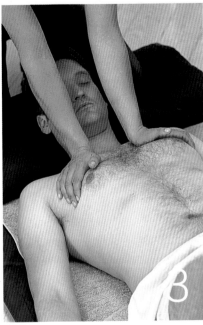

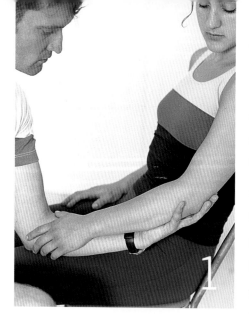

Tennis Elbow

As the name suggests, this complaint is associated with strenuous racket games such as tennis and is caused by untreated tightness and over-straining of the wrist extensors or by nodules and lesions that make the muscles prone to injury. The initial sign of tennis elbow is an ache not at the elbow but in the mid-section of the forearm, which may wear off but returns each time there is activity of the arm and wrist. In the worst case the wrist, not the elbow, needs to be immobilized for a period of time, but in most instances deep friction massage (see page 34) and manipulation of the joints will relieve the complaint.

1

Facing your partner, support their arm with your forearm and hold their elbow in your upturned, cupped hand.

2

Place your thumb on the outside of the elbow with your fingers underneath to apply counter pressure and, working around the outside of the elbow, apply pressure with the pad of your thumb, rotating it at the same time.

3

With your hands in the same position as for step 2, use the tip of your thumb instead of the pad to apply pressure by moving it backwards and forwards across the elbow in short strokes. Continue for one to two minutes, or to your partner's tolerance level, as this stroke can cause some discomfort.

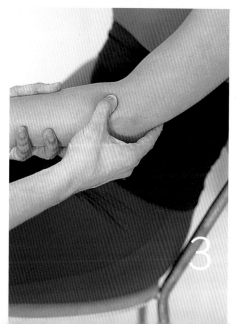

Golfer's Elbow

As with tennis elbow, the name describes a complaint suffered by people who play a particular sport, in this instance, golf. The causes are the same as for tennis elbow, but this time they relate to the upper arm. The symptoms are different from those of tennis elbow; the first sign of golfer's elbow being pain in the wrist joint when the elbow is extended and facing upwards. During activity, aching occurs between the elbow and shoulder in the upper arm.

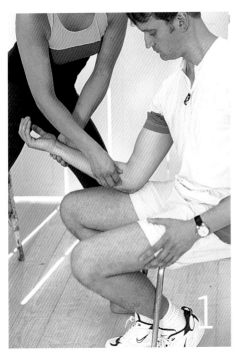

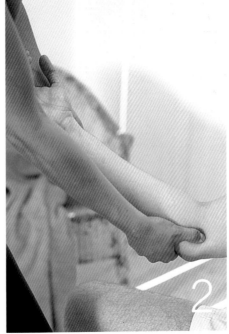

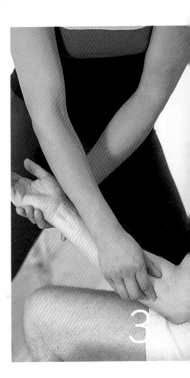

Tennis and Golf

The massages for golfer's elbow are essentially the same as for tennis, the only difference being that tennis elbow is treated on the outside of the elbow and golfer's elbow on the inside.

1

With your partner's arm facing upwards, make sure the elbow is supported either on their thigh or on a stable surface and support their wrist with your hand.

2

Place your thumb on the inside of the elbow and, working around the area, apply pressure with the pad of your thumb, rotating it at the same time.

3

With your hands in the same position as for step 2, use the tip of your thumb instead of the pad to apply pressure by moving it backwards and forwards across the inside of the elbow in short strokes. As this area can be very tender, continue only to your partner's comfort level.

Frozen Shoulder

If you have a pain in your shoulder as if you have slept awkwardly and then suddenly cannot lift your arm, and if every time you try, you feel an excruciating, deep burning pain and have no strength in your arm you have a frozen shoulder. This is caused by injury or repetitive exercise, and those over the age of 40 are more susceptible to the problem. The medical name is adhesive capsulitis. Each joint is surrounded by a capsule containing fluid to lubricate movement, and inflamed cells move into this capsule and cause parts of it to stick together, eventually 'freezing' the joint. The shoulder joint can become so frozen that some sufferers have less than ten per cent of their movement in any direction. Specialists stress the importance of early help, and one of the most effective treatments involves pressure and gradual stretching of the deep soft tissue and tendons.

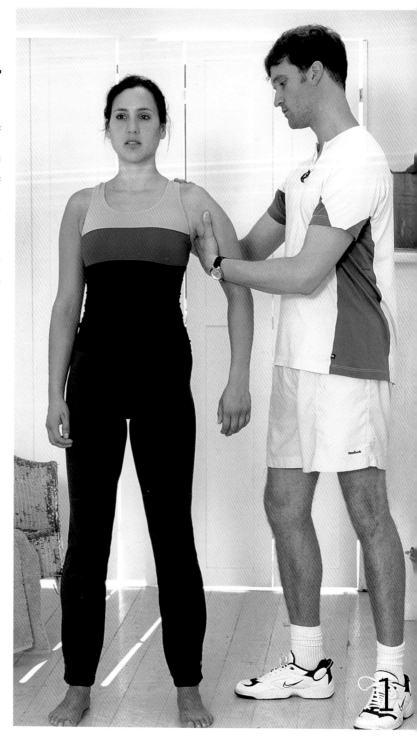

1

In a standing position, support your partner's upper arm with both hands and place one hand on the underside of the shoulder joint, lifting it very slightly. Move gently, as this can feel very tender or even painful to your partner.

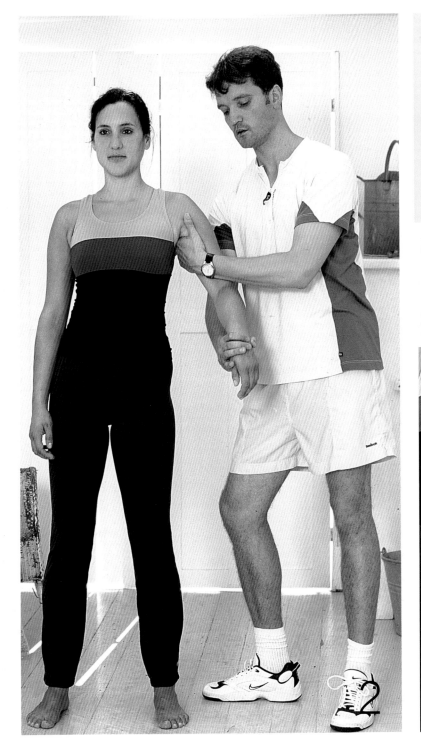

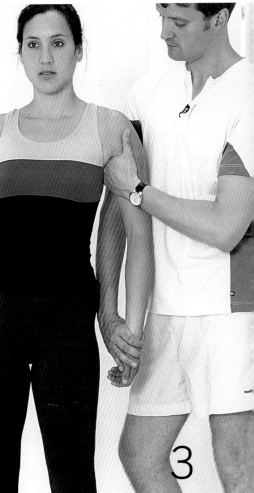

2

Keeping one hand under the arm, slide your other hand down to your partner's wrist for support and pull their straight arm forwards and outwards to a comfortable point of resistance.

3

Keeping your hands in the same position as in step 2, pull outwards with the hand under their shoulder, at the same time pulling down with the hand supporting their wrist. Hold the stretch for as long as your partner can tolerate, then release.

Rehabilitation

Massage of all types is one of the keys to a healthy body, and there are many self-help routines that can be applied to keep you supple and prevent injuries caused by playing sports and taking exercise or to strengthen your body following injury.

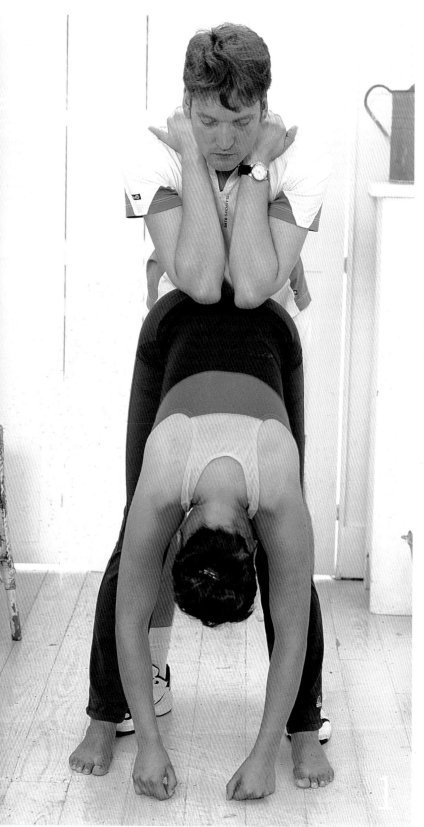

1

This position is taken from Hellerwork, a bodywork therapy that involves the stretching of tissues and an education in body awareness. It is good for relieving joint pains and releasing tension. Stand in front of your partner, both of you with feet hip width apart. With relaxed knees, drop your head and upper torso slowly downwards to a comfortable level, while your partner places their hands on either side of their neck with elbows resting on your lower back. They then apply pressure through their arms and elbows, and release. Repeat three to five times.

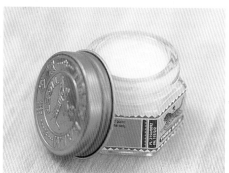

Tip

Tiger balm, made from natural ingredients, was once prepared for Chinese Emperors to soothe aches and pains. Today sports people often use it during massage to promote blood flow and for its mild analgesic properties.

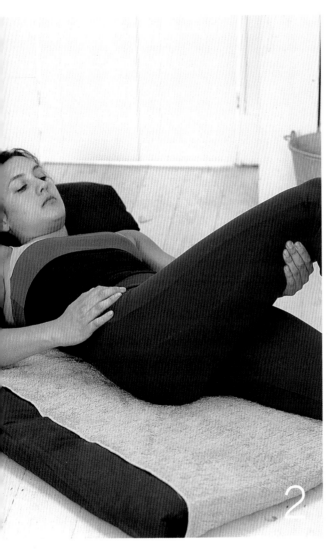

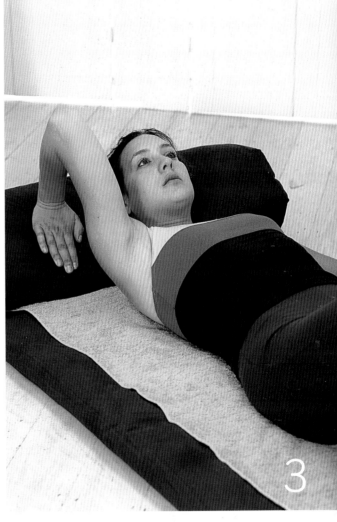

2

Lying comfortably face up with your head supported, place one hand on the underside of the opposite leg just above the knee joint and gradually pull the leg across the thigh of the other leg to a comfortable resistance point. Hold for five to ten seconds and relax. Repeat three to five times, then gently return to the starting point before moving to the other leg.

3

Keeping the starting position of step 2, lift your arm straight upwards to a vertical position, flex your elbow and lower your forearm back towards the side of your head, palm upwards, and hold at a comfortable point of resistance, then release. Repeat three to five times, then gently return to the starting point. Move to the other arm and repeat.

Body Alignment

Re-evaluating your posture and alignment together with massage can keep your body fresh and relaxed, thereby reducing tension. To create a stronger, stress-free spinal column means paying yourself more attention, and a simple routine of exercises carried out on a regular basis can help you to achieve this.

If you are prone to lower back tension, rounded shoulders and a forward-leaning head, this simple alignment technique can be done when your are standing or sitting down. It takes the pressure off the lower back, and if you practise it frequently your muscles can be trained to hold this renewed alignment without effort.

1

Find a door frame or a straight corner, place your feet with the heels touching the vertical surface and lean the whole of your body straight against the support with your arms at your side. Take a deep breath and press back with your whole torso so that there is no gap between you and the support, then breathe out, holding the position. Imagine you have a string at the top of your head pulling you upwards. Repeat this on a regular basis, daily or weekly.

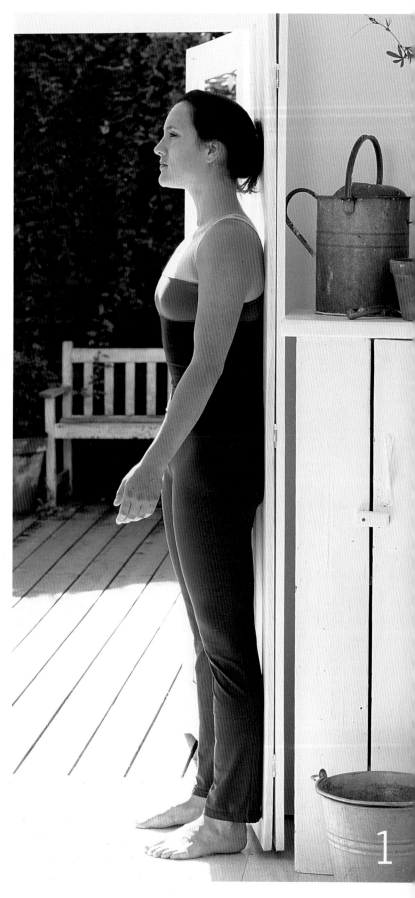

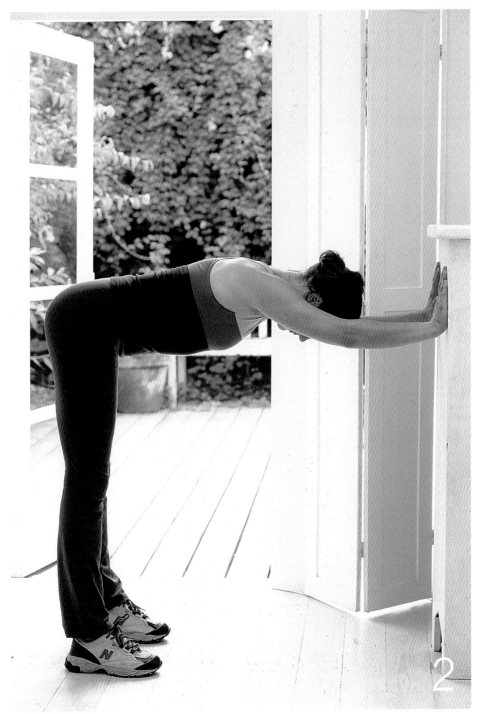

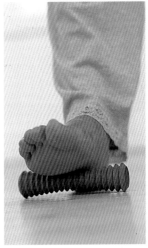

Tip

Structural problems of the feet, such as a high arch, will improve significantly with massage; work vigorously for a fallen arch and slowly to relax a high arch.

2

Find a hip-high surface or something stable to lean on, stand an arm's length away with your feet hip width apart and slowly lower your upper torso with arms outstretched until your back is flat and at right angles to your legs. With legs and arms straight, push yourself against the support surface and hold the position for three to five minutes or as long as it feels comfortable, then release. Return to the upright position slowly, bending your knees as you do so. Repeat three times, once or twice a day.

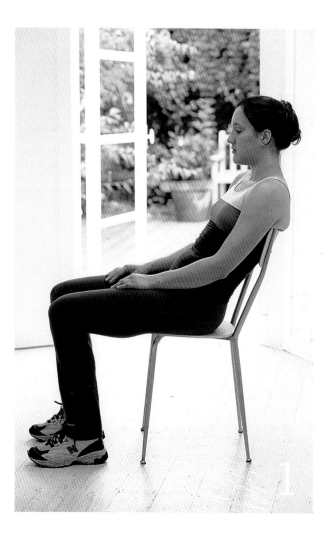

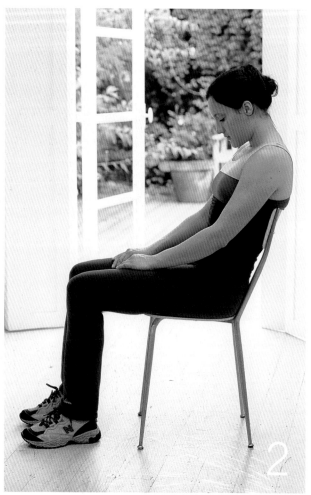

1

The normal position most people adopt when they sit is with a gap between the lower back and the chair, with the head slightly bowed.

2

To realign your body, pull your chin in slightly (not up or down), with the top of the back of your head pulled straight up. Visualize your shoulders dropping back and down. Breathe in and tighten your abdominal muscles, pushing your lower back into the chair, and breathe out.

3

In this new realigned position, place your hands on your shoulders and move your elbows back slightly, in line with your torso, breathe in at the same time and hold for five to ten seconds. Release and repeat.

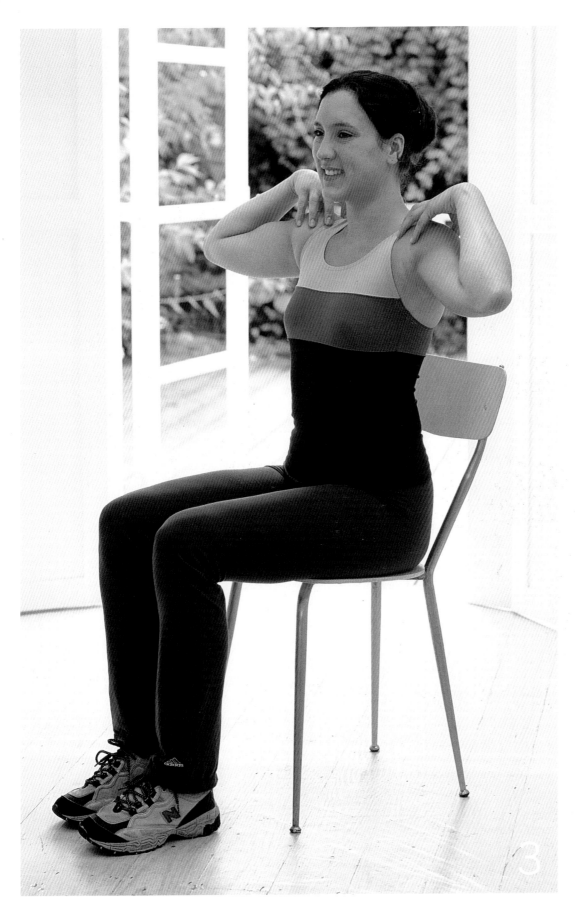

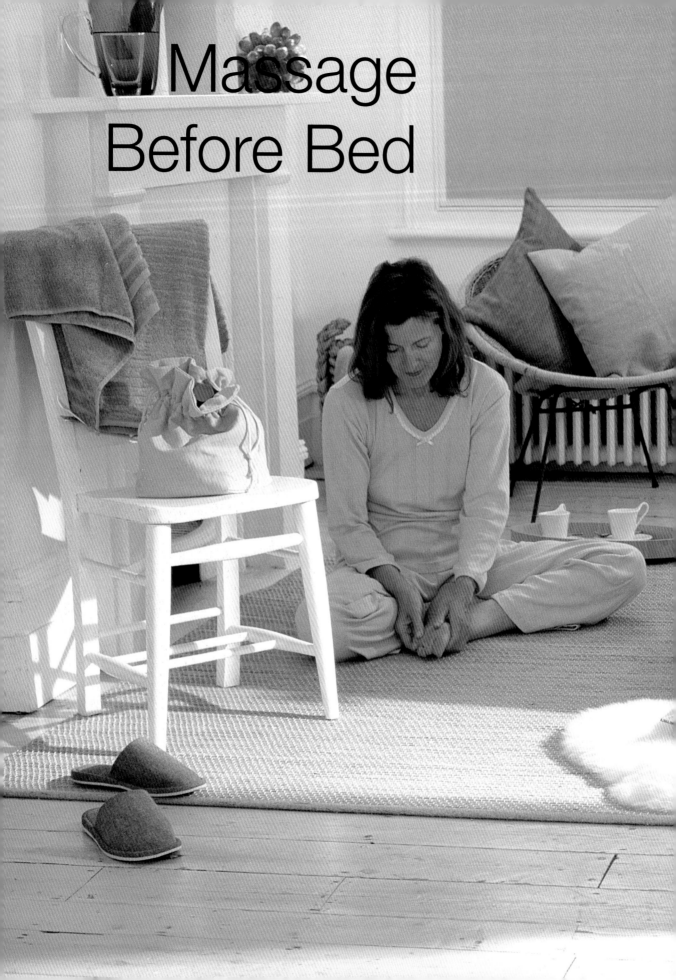

Massage
Before Bed

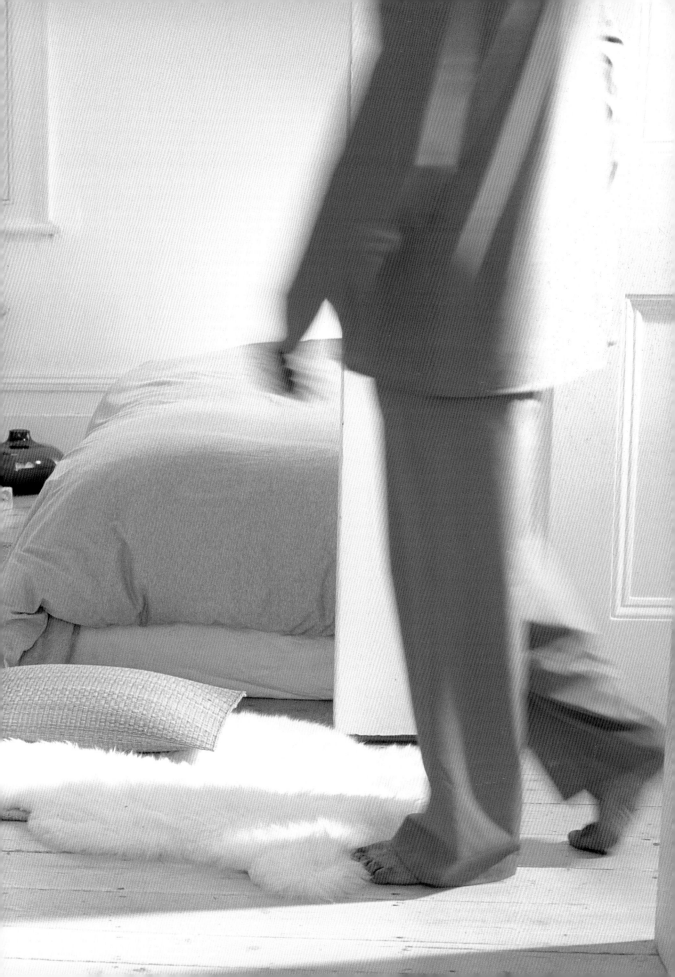

Relax the Muscles and Ease the Joints

Just before going to bed is an ideal time to enjoy a deep, relaxing massage. Take a long, warm bath or shower beforehand to help relax the muscles that have been working hard all day. As we get older, all the symptoms of adult life – tensions from long, stressful days in the office, overworked muscles from physical labour or aches and stiffness caused by sedentary employment – rise to the surface and all can benefit from massage. At the same time, massage is also a channel for communication with your partner and is as therapeutic to give as it is to receive. Enhance your massage with the use of pre-blended oils to suite your mood and encourage a good night's sleep.

Lower Legs

This routine will promote relaxation of the calf, improve circulation and help to eliminate toxins from the body.

1

Position yourself at the foot of your partner, then ask them to flex their knee and rest the top of their foot on your shoulder. Cup your hands on either side of the calf muscles one above the other and use petrissage strokes (see page 30) to apply even pressure, squeezing in opposite directions between your fingers and the heels of your hands, then release. Repeat three to five times.

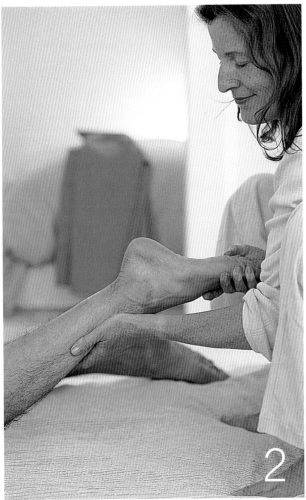

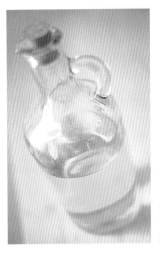

Tip

For an especially soothing bedtime massage use a pre-blended oil containing a few drops of a calming oil, such as lavender or chamomile, to encourage a good night's sleep.

2

Gently take your partner's foot from your shoulder and hold it in one hand, supporting the underside of the leg with the other hand. Place your thumb in the groove on the outer edge of the leg and effleurage (see page 28) down from above the ankle to the knee with pressure from your thumb and the flat of your hand. Lift off the pressure while remaining in contact and glide back to the starting position. Repeat three to five times.

3

Lower your partner's leg further, still supporting the ankle with one hand, and place your other hand palm down on the top of the calf. Effleurage from the ankle to the knee with pressure on the upward stroke, returning down the side of the leg. Repeat three to five times.

Move to the other leg and repeat steps 1–3.

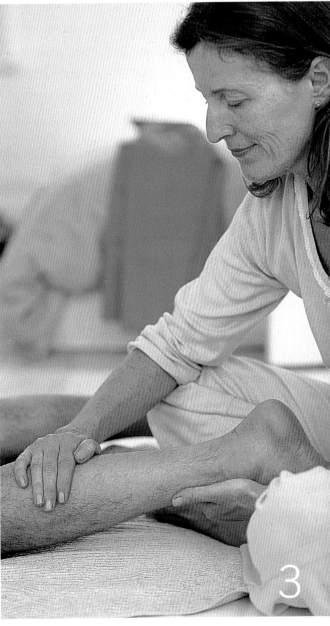

Back and Shoulders

These movements should release tension in the lower back area and help to mobilize the shoulders.

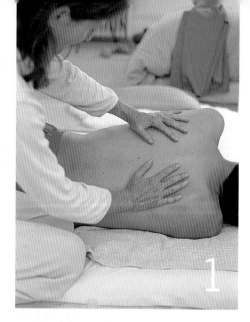

1

The back area is often like a suit of armour, held rigid in a protective mechanism throughout the day. To enable your partner to 'shed' this suit, position yourself to their side at about hip level and ask them to lie on their side with their back towards you. Make sure they are comfortable and well supported. Gently place the flat of both hands on either side of the spine on the lower back area and effleurage (see page 28) up towards the shoulders, returning down the sides of the torso, with pressure on the upward stroke. Repeat three to five times. This is the basic stroke that is used to warm up the area and apply the oil.

2

Place one hand on your partner's shoulder to maintain contact, then make a fist with the other and, using the knuckling stroke (see page 34), lean in and work up the back along the side of the spine to the shoulder, returning down the side of the torso with the flat of your hand. Repeat the stroke three to five times, then move to the other side of the spine and repeat the process.

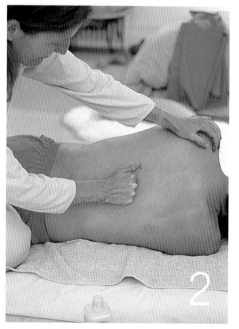

3

Using one hand, place your thumb on one side of the spine and your fingers on the other, so that the web of your hand straddles the vertebrae. Flex your thumb slightly and with the tip push up the back in 5cm (2in) long strokes until you have covered the whole area, gliding back with the flat of your hand to calm the area. Repeat the movement three to five times before moving to the other side.

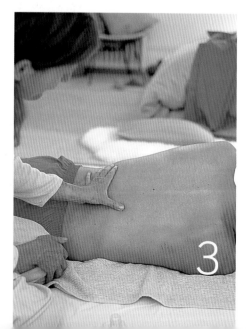

SAFETY FIRST

Remember: always work on either side of the spine, never directly over it.

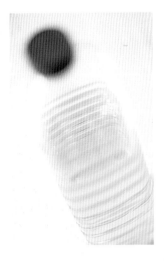

Tip

You do not have to buy special oil to be able to give a massage – a simple sunflower oil that you have in the storecupboard is suitable. Use it plain or add essential oils.

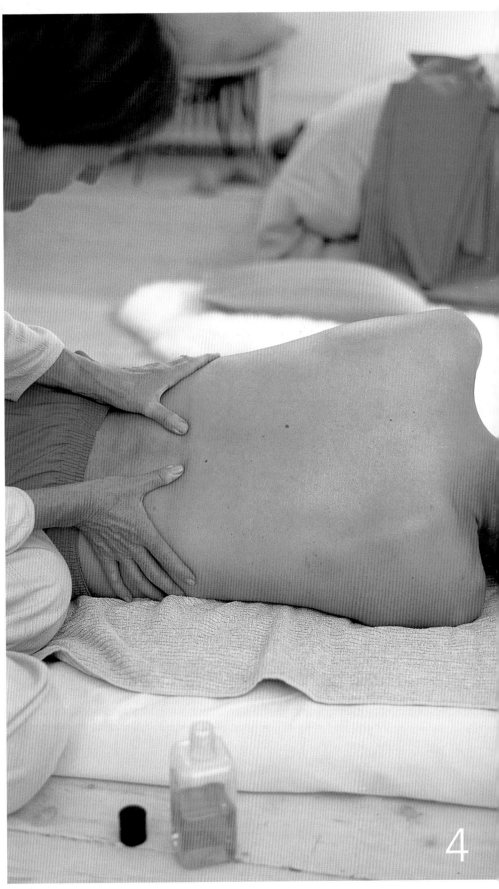

4

Place your thumbs on either side of the spine on the lower back and with the pads effleurage up the back to the shoulders, returning with a flat hand down the sides of the torso. Repeat three to five times.

Neck and Shoulders

Neck stiffness and shoulder aches will respond to this sequence.

1

With your partner lying in the same position as for the back and shoulders sequence (see pages 154–5), move around to face them. Supporting the front of the shoulder with one hand, place the flat of the other on the shoulder blade and, with pressure on the upward stroke, effleurage (see page 28) up over the area towards the base of the neck. Repeat three to five times.

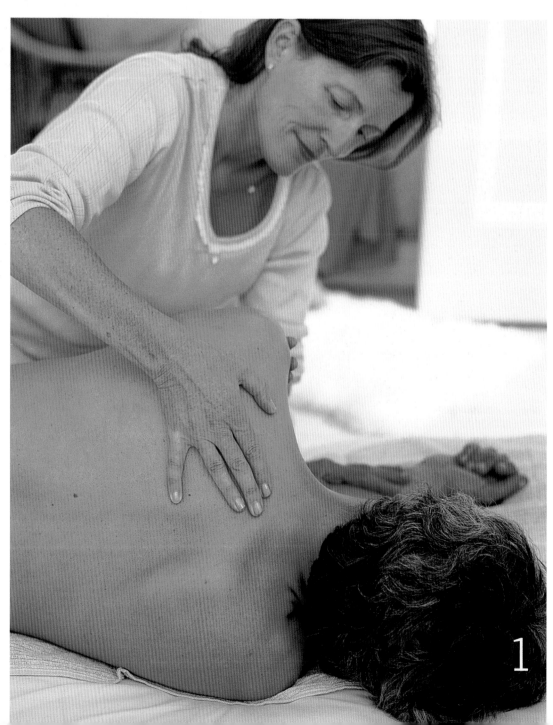

1

2

Place your hands palm down, one on the front of the shoulder joint and the other on the back, sandwiching the shoulder and the collarbone. Effleurage down towards the neck area, applying gentle pressure on the downward stroke and a slight pull on the return, to stretch the neck and shoulder muscles.

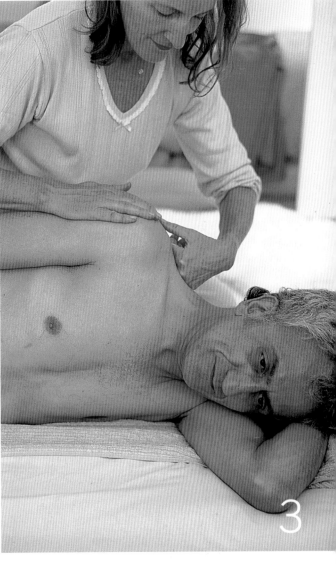

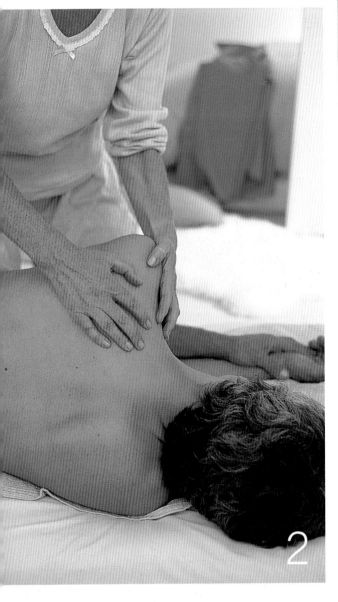

3

Once again working from behind, rest one hand on the top of the shoulder and make a fist with the fingers of the other hand. Place the flat of the fist, not the knuckles, at the base of the neck and, keeping flat to the surface, effleurage to the edge of the shoulder, then ease off the pressure, lift and return to the base of the neck. Adjust the pressure to the response of your partner to avoid discomfort. Repeat several times.

Ask your partner to lie on their opposite side and repeat steps 1–3.

Knees

Legs and knees often suffer from fatigue and sometimes swell in the evenings, as they have been carrying the heavy weight of our bodies all day. Busy parents and grandparents often never get the time to sit down until the children have gone to bed and it is time to retire for the evening. The following movements will help to mobilize the knee joints.

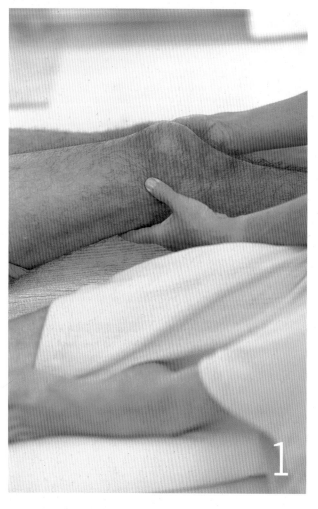

2

Asking your partner to flex their knee, take both hands and, using the pads of your fingers, effleurage in circular movements up and around the area. This will encourage blood flow around the knee, which in turn will ease tension and stiffness.

1

With your partner lying face up, position yourself to their side so that you can reach the knee area without overstretching. Place your hands on either side of the knee and gently effleurage (see page 28) around the area to ease and warm the joint.

3

Supporting one side of the knee, take the other and place your thumb just above the top of the joint. Using the pad, work upwards in a curved line using short strokes, gradually covering the whole of the area. This will help to disperse any toxins or fluid.

Repeat steps 1–3 several times until the joint feels mobilized, then move to the opposite leg and repeat the process.

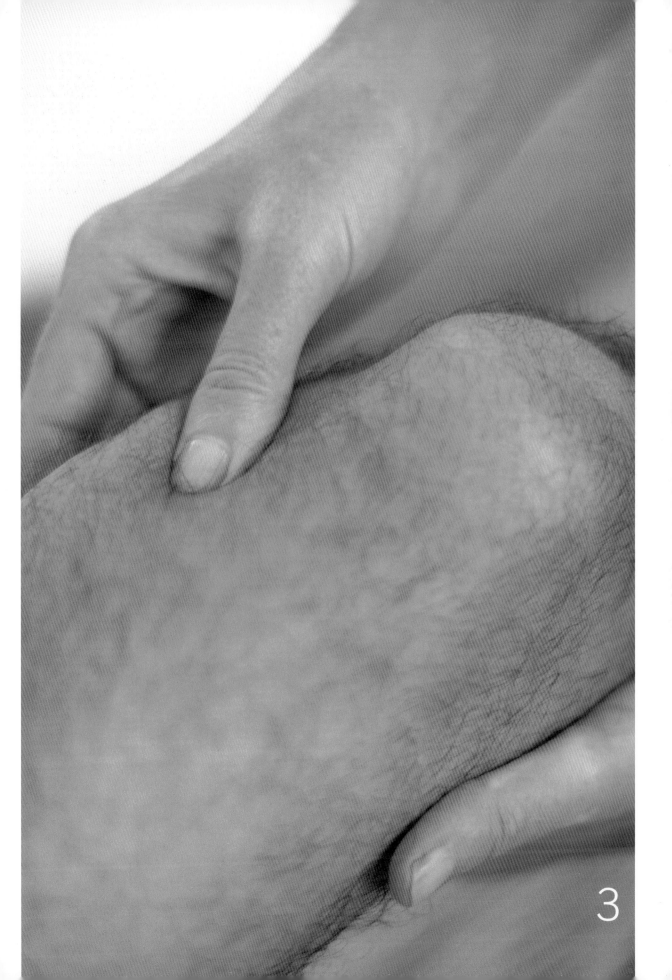

3

Thighs

The muscles in the thighs are usually overworked and need deeper work to break down the tensions and tightness. Climbing up and down stairs and walking on inclines will also leave the muscle at the back of the thigh feeling taut and sore.

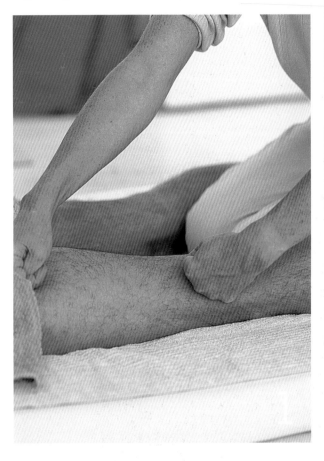

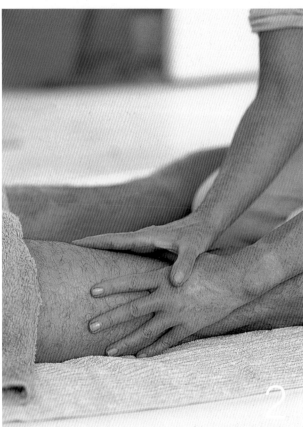

Tip

Before you start a massage make sure you have plenty of clean, soft towels close to hand. You can use them to keep your partner warm or to support individual limbs.

1

With your partner lying face down, position yourself between the legs at knee level. Make a fist with both hands and apply the knuckling stroke (see page 34) from the knee to the top of the thigh in a hand-over-hand manner, lifting off at the end of the stroke and returning the hands to repeat the stroke three to five times.

2

Place both hands flat down on the back of your partner's thigh, with one thumb on top of the other. Applying pressure with both thumbs, glide up the back of the thigh, returning with one hand on either side of the leg ready to repeat the stroke three to five times.

3

Move side-on to your partner, positioning yourself away from the leg on which you are working. Place both hands on the back of the thigh and apply the wringing stroke (see page 31), leaning inwards to apply firm pressure. Moving the hands in opposite directions and in a continuous rhythmic movement, work across the whole of the area.

Move to the other leg and repeat steps 1–3.

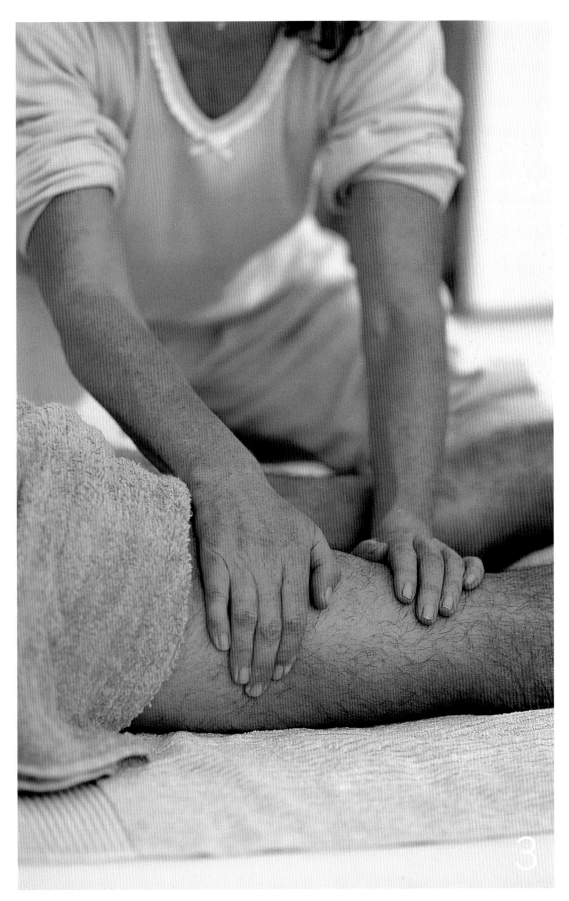

3

Feet

The sole of the foot contains thousands of nerve endings and connects to other parts of the body with reflexes, and most people love having their feet massaged because it affects the whole of the body. The feet are very complex parts of our anatomy and act as the body's shock absorbers. Apart from general tiredness as a result of carrying our body around, tension may occur in the ball of the foot due to high arches or, more superficially, footwear with high heels.

1

With yourself and your partner in a comfortable position, take the foot in both hands with the sole facing you. Wrap your fingers around the top of the foot and place your thumb on the ball. Using the whole length of your thumbs, apply pressure and pull the thumbs in opposite directions out towards the edge of the foot, lift off and return, ready to repeat. Work all across the length and width of the ball of the foot.

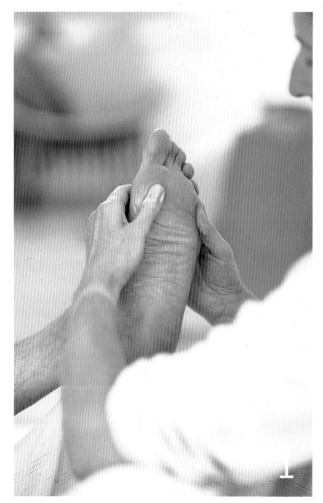

2

Supporting the heel and ankle firmly in one hand, with the thumb of your other hand massage using the thumb pads in a circling stroke, starting at the heel and ending just under the toes. Wrap the fingers of your working hand around the top of the foot for extra support and to counterbalance the pressure.

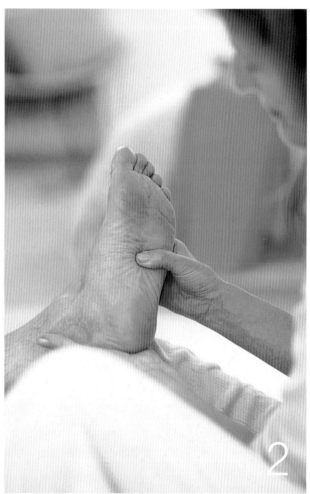

3

This is a wonderful stroke with which to finish off and to make your partner feel the massage is complete. Place your hands on the top and underneath of the foot and, with a very gentle effleurage stroke (see page 28), glide down from the ankle and, leaning back slightly, pull off over the toes. Repeat several times.

Move to the other foot and repeat steps 1–3.

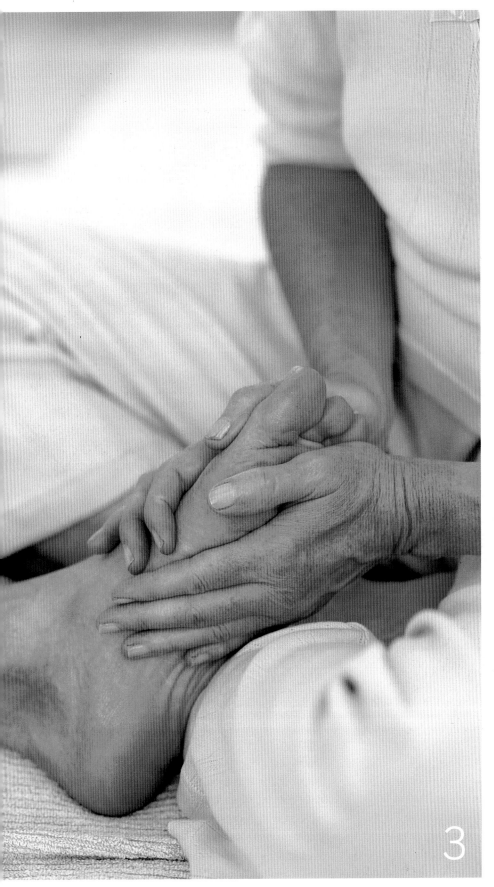

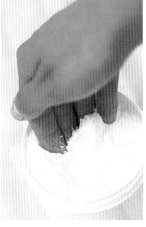

Tip

As an alternative to massage oil use a soothing peppermint foot lotion or a rich cream for a more luxurious feel. This will have the added benefit of moisturizing dry skin, which is common on this area of the body.

When you are massaging the feet, it is important that you apply a firm touch so that you do not tickle your partner.

3

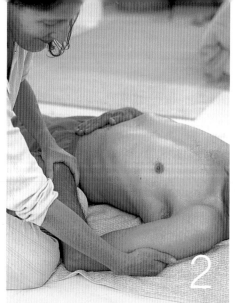

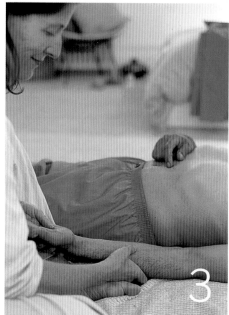

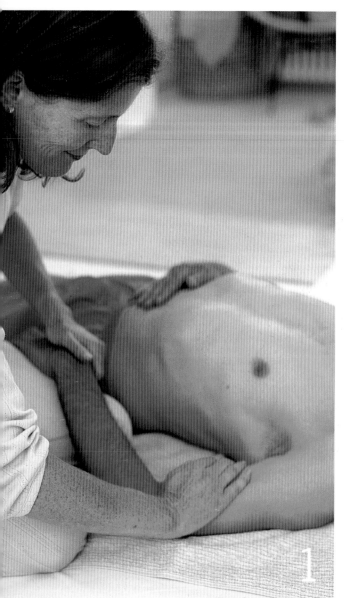

Arms and Hands

Arm massage is great for releasing pent-up emotions. This part of the body is very expressive – we show love by stroking and embracing in a very instinctive way. Use these strokes as a channel of communication between yourself and your partner.

1

Take your partner's hand in yours in a handshake-type clasp, and with the flat of your other hand effleurage (see page 28) up the arm from the wrist to the shoulder, lifting off the pressure slightly over the elbow joint.

2

When you reach the top of the arm, glide over the shoulder and return down the underside of the arm to your starting position. Repeat three to five times.

3

Still clasping the hand, place your thumb across the inner wrist and squeeze up from the wrist to the elbow, rocking forward at the same time, then glide back with no pressure. Repeat three to five times. You may find your partner's fingers opening and closing, as the muscles that control the fingers are located in the forearm.

4

Move to the upper arm and, using the petrissage stroke
(see page 30), squeeze the muscle between your fingers
and the heel of your hand, working up its length and
'milking' all the tension out of the area. Repeat three to
five times, then soothe over with an effleurage stroke.

Move to the other arm and repeat steps 1–4.

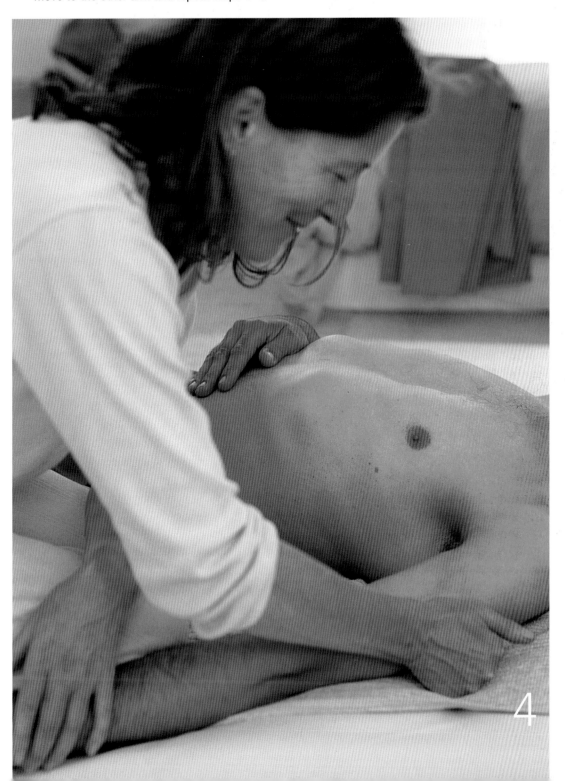

4

Insomnia and Anxiety

Insomnia is a side effect of stress and is usually linked with anxiety about something in our lives. Massage promotes sleep naturally, which is very important in breaking the cycle of fatigue. The ideal time to massage is just before retiring to bed, and an essential oil such as lavender can be used to enhance the benefits of the massage. Use gentle, rhythmic strokes or a face routine as shown here, and encourage your partner to let go of the thoughts of the day, empty their mind and drift.

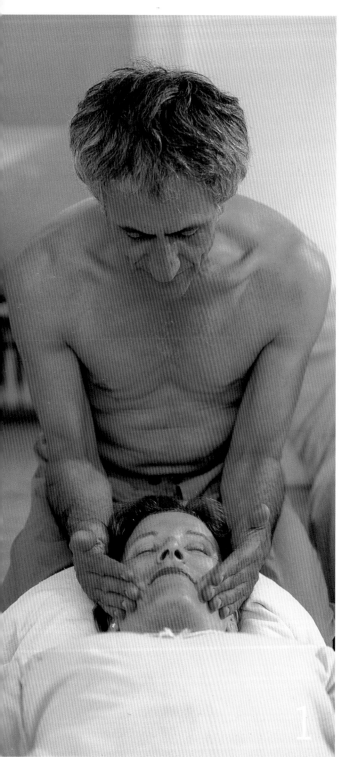

1

Making sure your partner is comfortable and warm, position yourself at their head and, leaning forward, place the fingers of both hands on the chin. With your finger pads rotating in small circles, move along around the jawline to just in front of the ear lobe. This is a very slow movement to expel the tension that is so often stored in this part of the face.

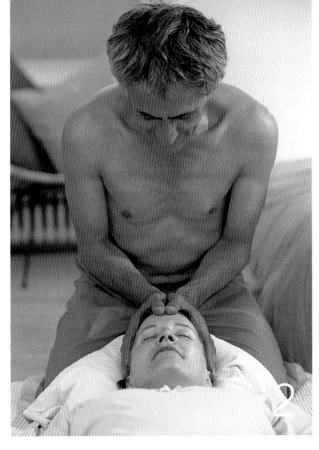

2

Place your thumbs together and flat to the surface at the centre of the forehead, holding the sides of the head. Glide each thumb outwards to the temples, lift off and return to the centre. Repeat several times, moving up over the whole of the forehead to the hairline.

3

Place your thumbs on top of each other at the centre of the forehead near the hairline, then exert pressure, hold for a few seconds and release. Repeat, moving up over the head to the centre.

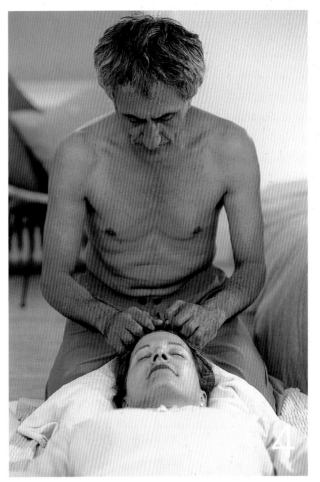

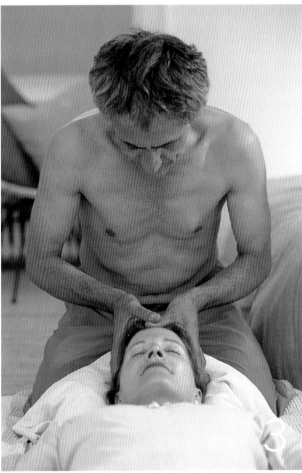

4

Draw the splayed fingers of both hands very slowly through your partner's hair in a combing action, moving one hand and then the other in a continuous, rhythmic motion.

Head, Neck and Shoulders

Often the most relaxing part of a massage, work on the head, neck and shoulders deserves special attention as it is frequently here that we build up excessive tension, because feelings of emotion and anger result in a tightening of the neck and throat. Take time with the strokes and give the massage with care and good thoughts.

1

Position yourself at your partner's head and make sure you are comfortable, as any slight movement will be transferred to your partner during this sequence. Turning your partner's head slightly away from the side you are massaging and with the other hand on the shoulder for contact, start at the top of the neck and glide your hand downwards using the effleurage stroke (see page 28) to the edge of the shoulder. Turn your hand slightly to return, scooping up the neck with the web of your hand. Repeat three to five times, then move to the other side of the neck and repeat.

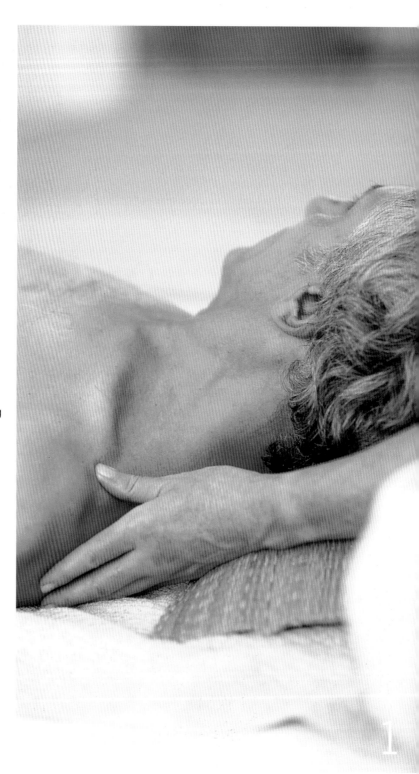

2

Cupping your hands over your partner's ears with your fingers wrapped underneath, use the heel of your hands to pull slowly downwards over the ears and off. Make sure the stretch is not so strong as to become uncomfortable. Repeat several times.

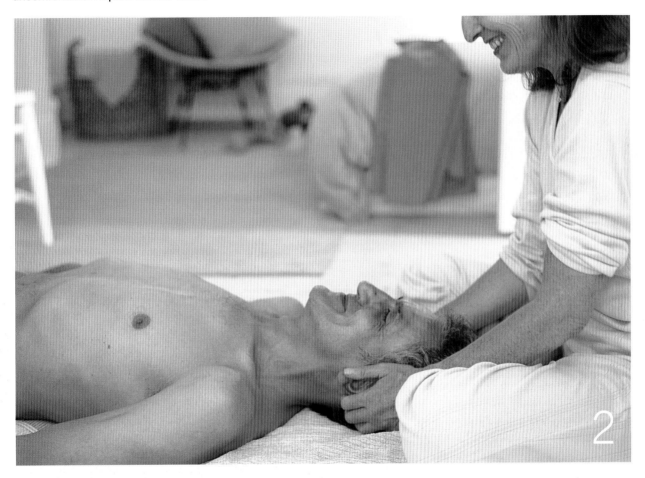

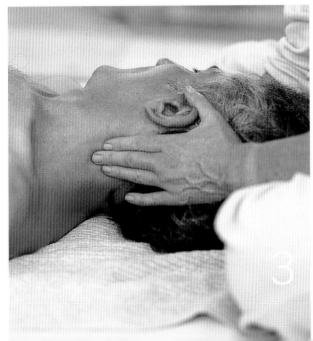

3

In order to turn your partner's head in a safe and confident way, hold it on either side with your thumbs above the ears and fingers behind in a V shape, lift very slightly and rest it on one hand that is cupped slightly. Make sure that you do not pull any hair and that your partner feels comfortable, as you want them to relax into your hands and not resist in order for the muscles to relax.

4

With your partner's head turned slightly away from the side being massaged, position the pads of your fingers along the base of the skull, press upwards and slowly rotate your fingers in very tiny circles. Work along the area, cradling the rest of the head in your hands.

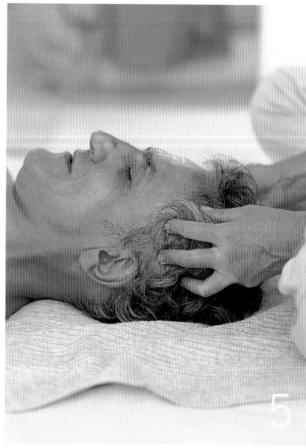

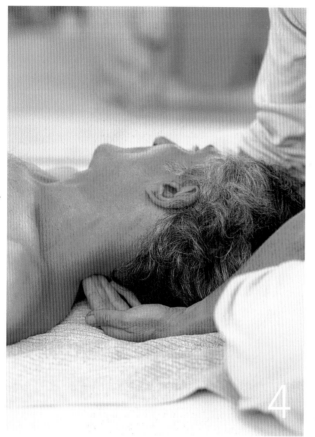

5

Using your fingers on either side of the head, press into the scalp and, in a 'shampooing' motion, work thoroughly over the whole head in a continuous, rhythmic movement. If you find this position difficult, use one hand only, remembering to keep contact with the other.

6

Move to a side position facing your partner, place your hands firmly over the tops of the shoulders and pull firmly towards you with the flat of your fingers. This is a gentle shoulder pull and should not raise the torso off the massage surface.

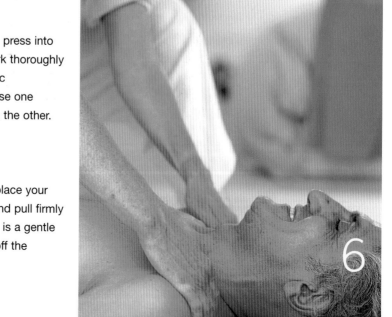

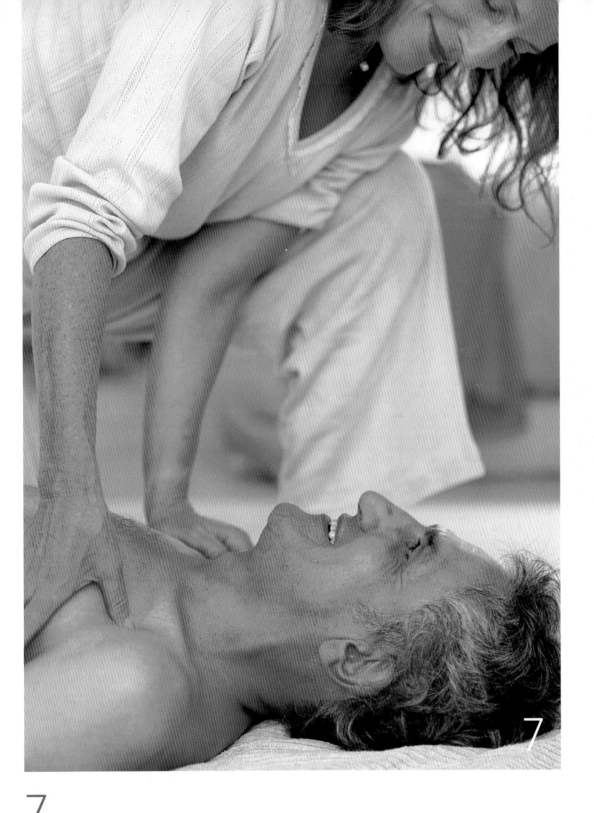

7

7

To release and relax this area further, with one hand resting on a
shoulder place the other on the pectoral muscle at the front of the chest.
With your thumb and the web of your hand, glide across the muscle to
the outer edge. Repeat two or three times, then move to the other side
and repeat.

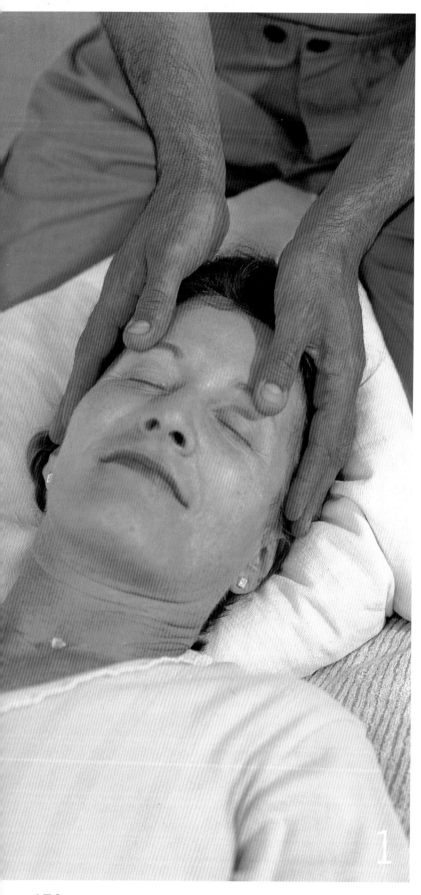

Face

Most massage to the face is based on shiatsu, which means 'finger pressure' in Japanese. Instead of long strokes, acupressure points are used to balance the body's energy. Gentle enough to relax, the pressure should feel firm but also caressing. We reflect tension and stress in our face with a tightening of the brow and jaw; calm and relaxation shows as a very 'open' face. Massaging the face enables us to drop some of our facial 'masks' and leads to a sense of deep relaxation. You may not need to use oil unless the skin is very dry or mature, when a very tiny amount will prevent you dragging the skin as you work.

SAFETY FIRST

Before you begin any face massage, make sure your partner is not wearing contact lenses.

1

Make contact by resting the flats of your thumbs next to each other on the centre of the forehead. Glide the flat of each thumb across the forehead to the outer edge, lift off and return, working the whole area from the hairline to brow.

2

Taking care, glide the thumbs across the eyebrows, working from the inner brow outwards and off at the sides of the head. Repeat three to five times. This movement soothes the whole of the eyebrow area.

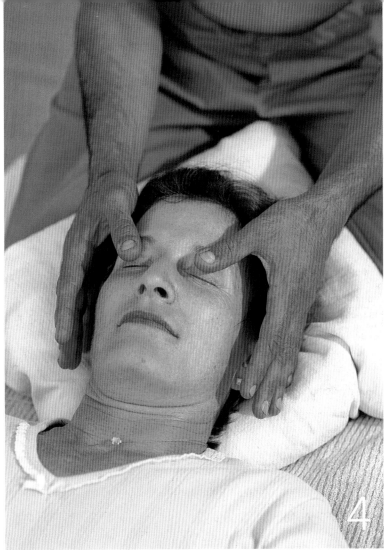

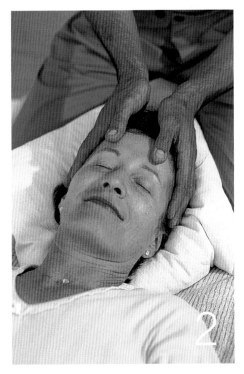

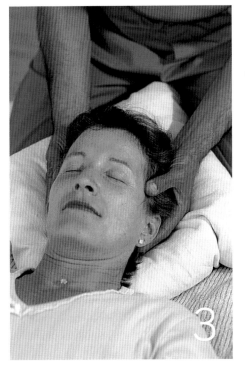

3

Place the pads of your thumbs on your partner's temples, resting in the natural hollow. With your fingers supporting the head behind the ears, make tiny circles over the temples. Alternatively, keep the thumbs stationary and press inwards, hold for a few seconds and release. This is an excellent remedy for tension and headaches.

4

Ask your partner to close their eyes, if they have not already done so. Bringing you thumbs inwards, start at the corner of the eye and carefully and lightly glide over the eyelids to the outer edge, then return. Repeat two or three times. If the eyes are too sensitive, or your partner is too nervous, do the stroke but without making contact.

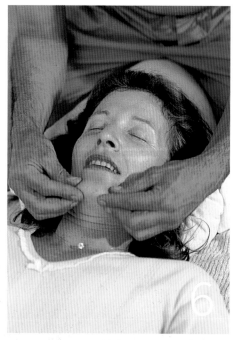

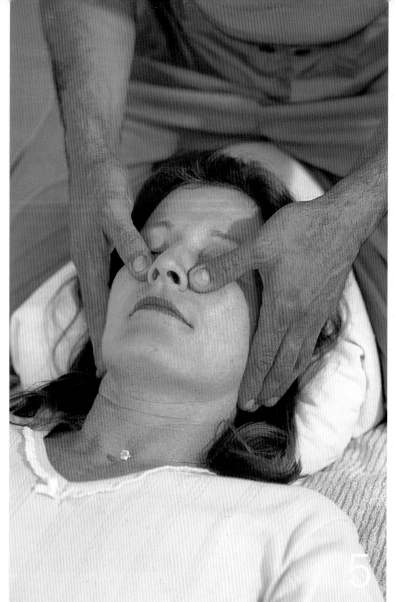

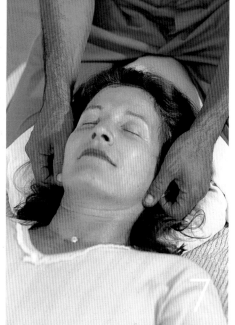

5

Starting from the top of the nostril, glide the tip of each thumb alongside the nose, sweep along the top of the cheekbone to the outer edge, pull off and return. Repeat once or twice. This stroke follows the path of the sinuses and will help release any congestion (see also page 62).

6

Place your thumbs and fingers on either side of the jawline at the centre and, in a rotation movement, work each hand slowly outwards towards the ears. You may notice that as the jaw relaxes your partner's mouth will open slightly, as a reflex to the massage and a sign that the tension held there is releasing.

7

When you reach the ears, with your whole thumb pull down gently and off at the edges. This is a very pleasurable stroke – Eastern philosophies believe that the ear is connected to and represents the whole of the body, so with this small movement your partner may feel relaxed all over.

8

Take the ears between your fingers and thumbs and gently pull outwards, stretching them away from the head. Then squeeze all around the lobes, holding for a few seconds before breaking contact.

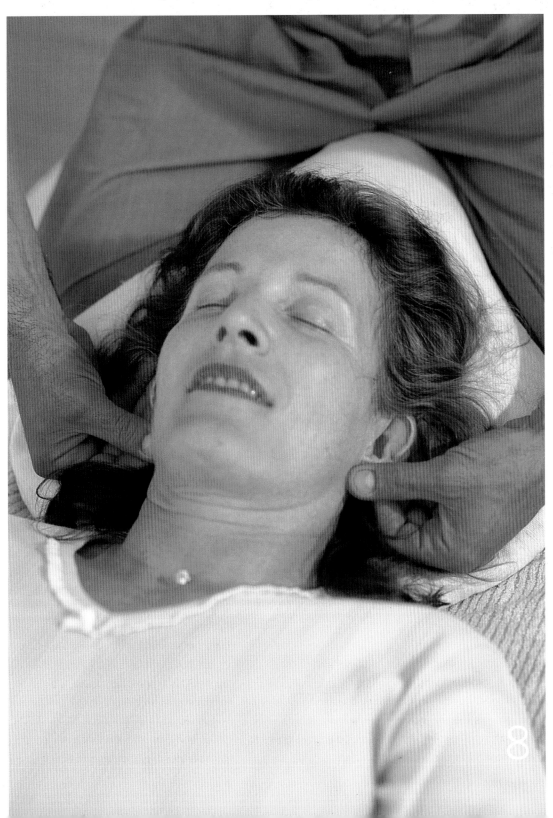

9

Move to the top of the head at hairline level and run your hands through your partner's hair, making sure that the tops of your fingers brush the whole of the scalp from front to back.

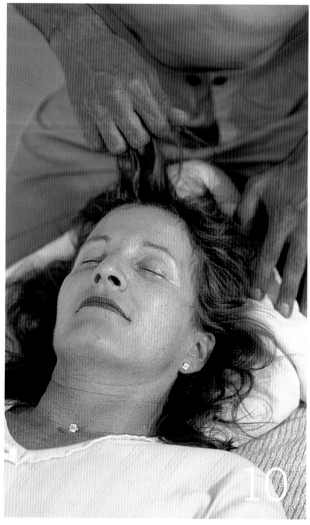

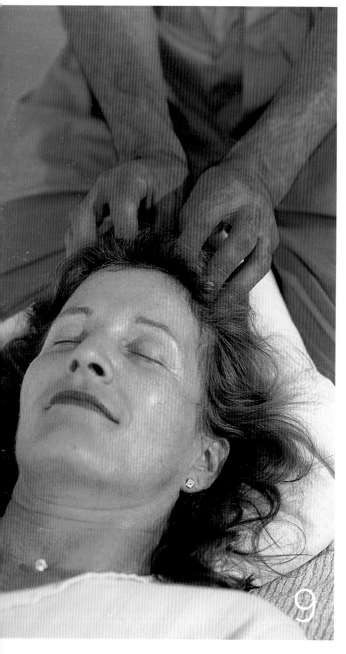

10

Take small strands of hair at a time and pull towards you very gently, working in sections over the whole of the head.

11

By now your partner should almost have drifted off and will be ready for bed. To finish, place the flat of one hand across the whole of the forehead with the other hand on top and hold for five to ten seconds.

Happy Ending

Your partner should now be feeling total contentment and completeness. You can see this reaction by reading your partner's facial expression. You, too, should be feeling very relaxed, as this routine is very calming and therapeutic.

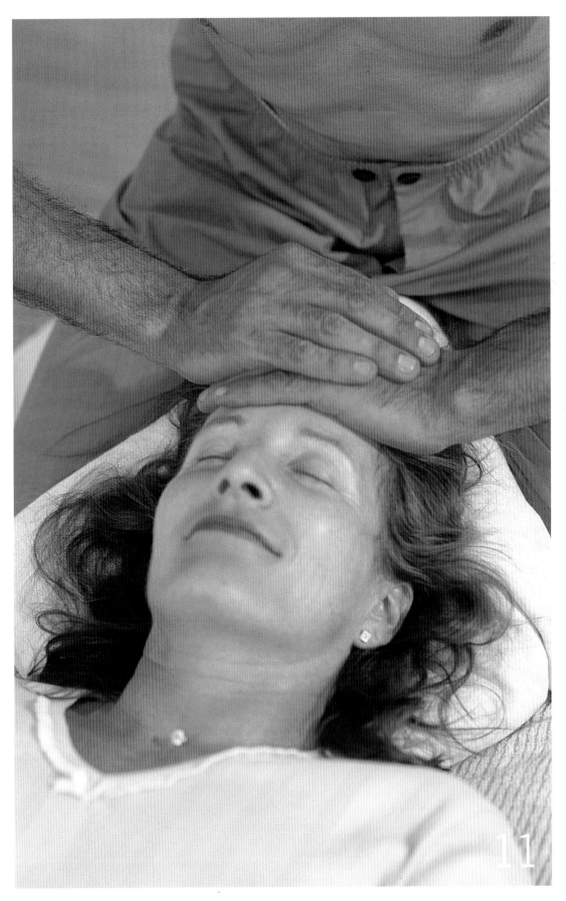

11

Sensual Massage

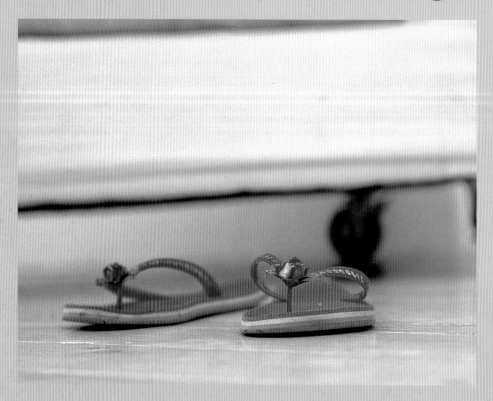

With the right environment, touch and aromas, massage can be a shared experience that helps couples to communicate better and devote time to each other in otherwise busy lives. Book a date in your diaries with each other, turn off the television and your mobile phones, shut out any distracting noise and set the scene by giving your partner your undivided attention.

To create a perfect atmosphere combine soft lighting, candles, scents and flowers with your favourite relaxing music. Remember that the evening is for both of you, so make sure your choice of aromas and music is mutually enjoyable. Have some massage aids (see pages 40–1 and 188–9) to hand.

Massage puts both of you in touch with something quite magical that would normally escape your day-to-day awareness of each other. It enables you to sense where and how to touch, and for how long. Let instinct guide your hands, and make sure that you are both open to the flow of love and tenderness between giver and receiver. Use a sensual blend of massage oils to enhance your mood: the scents activate the body's limbic system (part of the brain concerned with emotion, hunger and sex) and are a must if you want your partner to emerge from the massage in the mood for love.

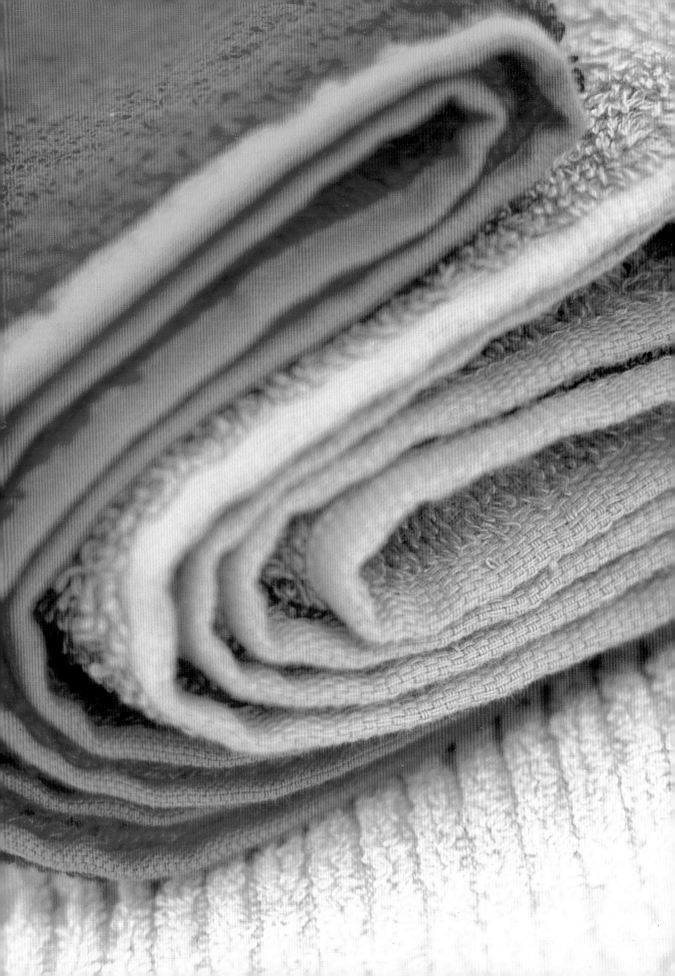

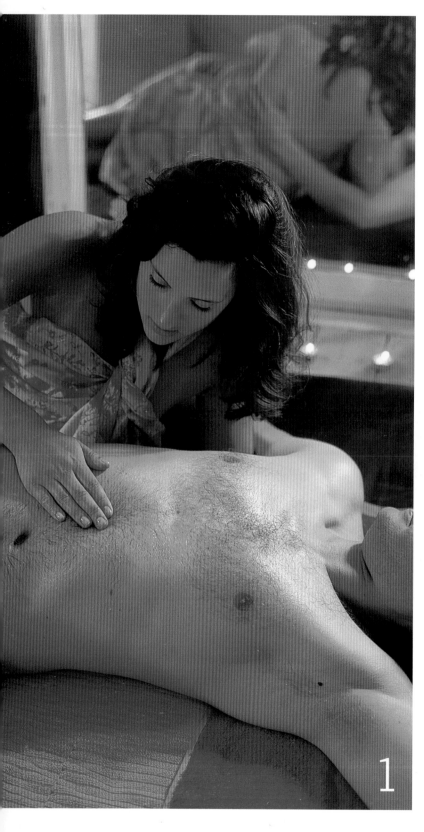

Stomach

This is where we often hold all of our emotions and is a special area, so treat it with care.

1

With your partner face up, lie to the side of them in a comfortable position and place the flat of one hand on their navel. With the effleurage stroke (see page 28) moving in a clockwise direction, make ever-widening circles, gradually covering the area from the ribcage to the lower abdomen. For this sensual massage, much lighter, pleasurable strokes are used so as not to break the mood.

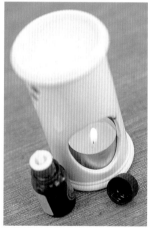

Tip

Enhance the soft light provided by candles by using them in special holders that also contain essential oils, which release their aroma as they are warmed.

Underarms

Every part of the body has the potential for arousal, so start with the least obvious parts first.

1

One of the body's erogenous zones, the underarms are often neglected in general massage. Lying in the same position as for the stomach massage (see opposite), sweep the flat of your hand up from the stomach diagonally to the underarm area, using a long effleurage stroke.

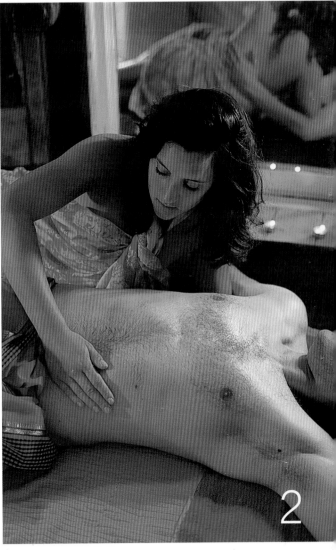

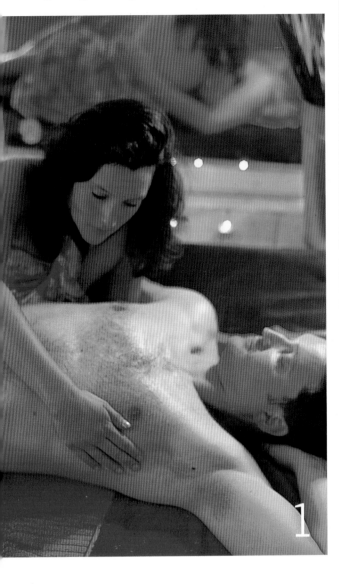

2

Return down the side of the torso. Use plenty of massage oil and repeat steps 1 and 2 several times in a continuous, flowing movement. Combine a light, feathery touch with firmer strokes, making your fingers 'dance' with your partner.

Move to the other side and repeat the process.

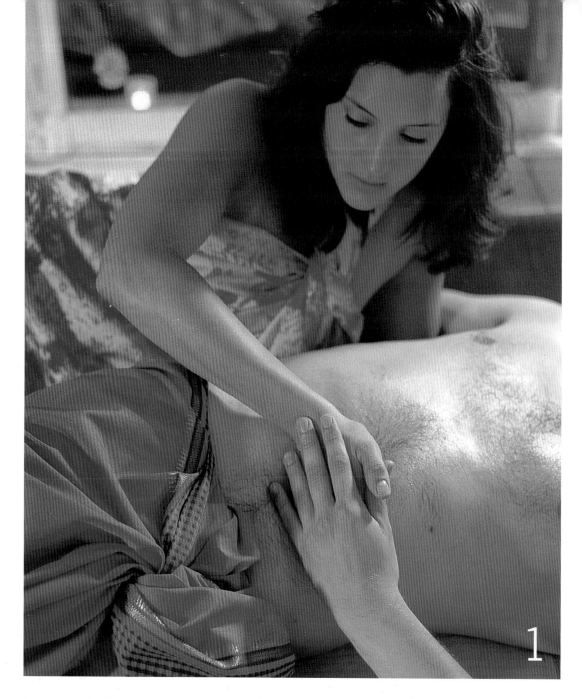

Lower abdomen

The skin, the body's largest organ, is made up of millions of sensory receptors, which can be stimulated in a more sensual and erotic way by enhancing simple touch. The lower abdomen is just one of the erogenous zones.

1

Place your partner's hand on top of yours, interlinking thumbs, and circle clockwise with the effleurage stroke (see page 28) over the lower abdomen. Go as low as you both feel comfortable – as your hands are linked, your partner can guide you to where they would like the massage stroke to reach.

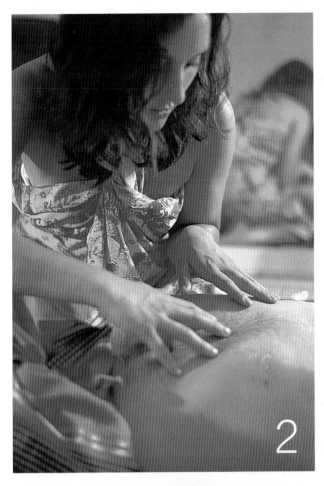

2

Moving to a position from which you can place both hands on your partner's abdomen, use the feathering stroke (see page 38) to work horizontally across the whole area. Be aware of your partner's breathing patterns as the abdomen rises and falls.

3

Returning to the side, use the same feathering technique to work vertically across the whole area. Take care to find the right balance of pressure to tease but not tickle.

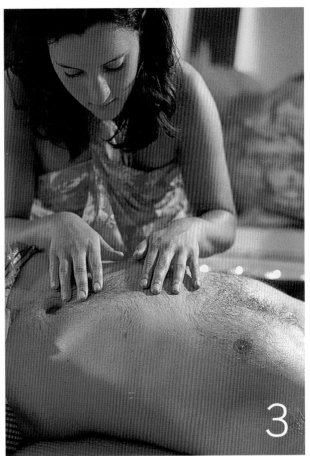

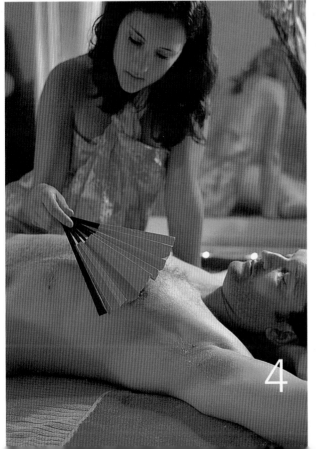

4

The skin is full of nerve endings and receptors that are stimulated by massage. Here we have used a fan to achieve a different sensation, but you could use anything suitable whose feel you and your partner enjoy. Simply stroke it lightly all over the lower abdomen and up the body to the chest area.

Thighs

Use the fingertips, the palms or even the back of the hands, change locations, rhythm and pace in an exploratory way. This position allows you to remain in eye contact and enjoy interaction with each other if you wish.

1

With your partner lying face up, position yourself so that their thighs are resting on your knees for support. Place one hand on each corresponding thigh just above the knee, and with the effleurage stroke (see page 28) glide down the top of the thigh, working on both legs simultaneously.

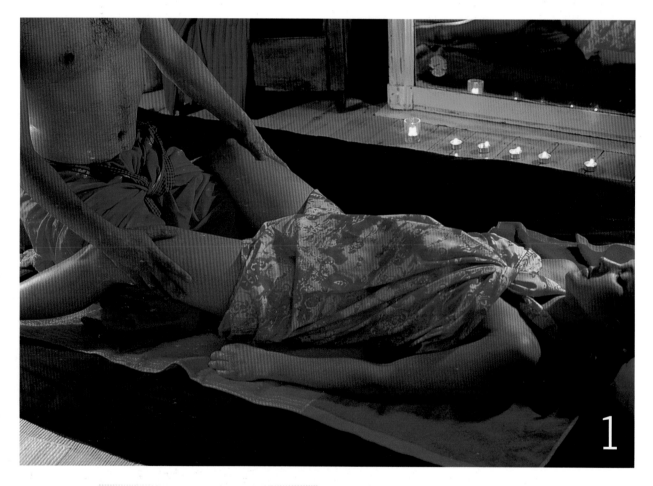

1

INNER THIGH MASSAGE

If you feel very comfortable with your partner, this sequence can be applied to the erogenous zone of the inner thigh from the same position. Make sure you use plenty of oil or cream, as the skin is very soft here and should not be dragged.

2

When you reach the top of the thigh, move your hands outwards to the underside of the leg.

3

Return with the flat of your hand under the leg, back to the knee. Repeat steps 1–3 several times.

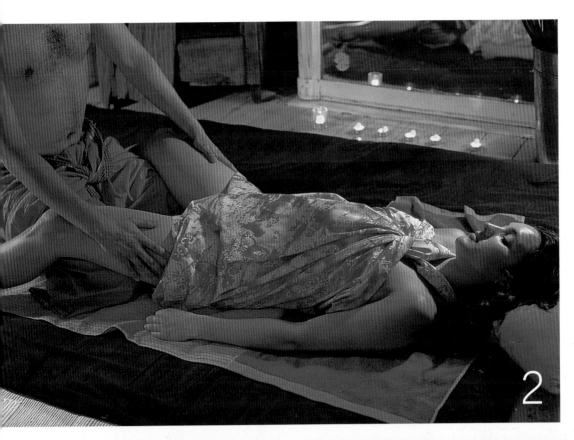

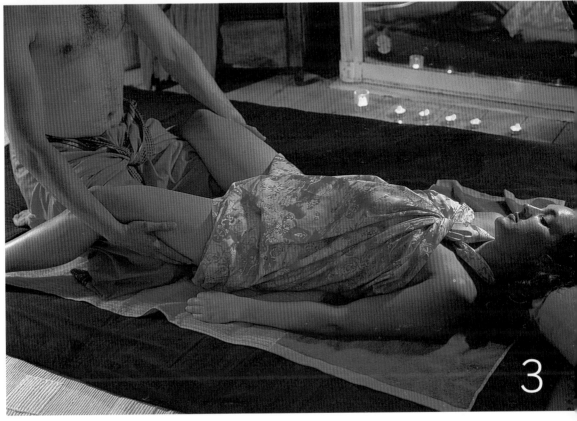

Back

Often a seat of tension and discomfort, the lower back is linked to problems connected with security and sexuality, so the more self-confidence a person has in these areas of life the less lower back pain they are likely to experience.

SAFETY FIRST

Remember: always work on either side of the spine, never directly over it.

1

With your partner lying face down, position yourself at their head. This is a great position from which to breathe against their skin or whisper sweet nothings in their ear. Place your hands palm down at the top of the centre shoulder, on either side of the spine.

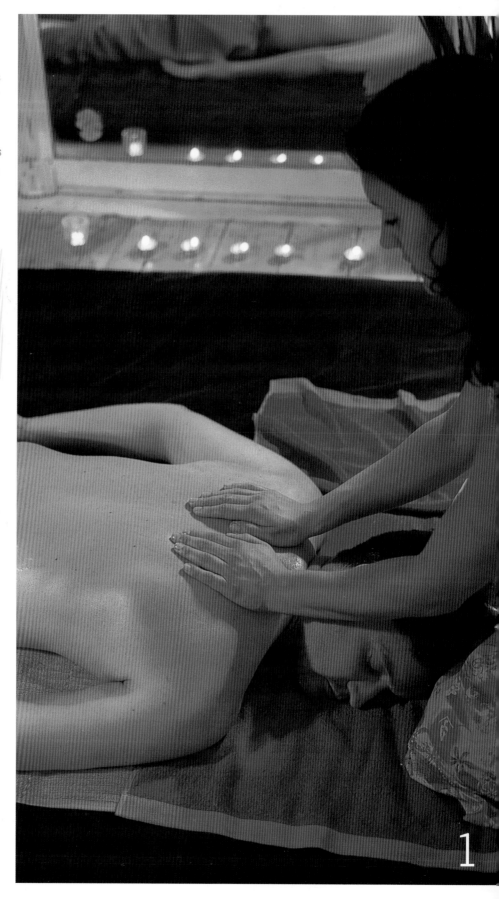

1

2

Glide down the back on either side of the spine using the effleurage stroke (see page 28). Stop at a comfortable reach, but if possible stroke as far as the top of the buttock area.

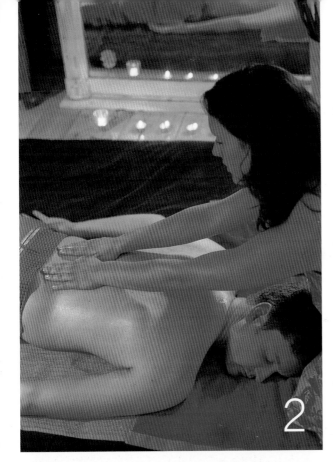

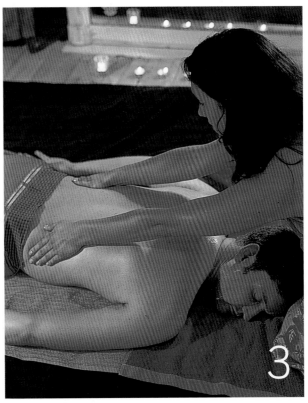

3

Sweep your hands in opposite directions outwards towards the sides of the torso and return up the sides with a slight pulling motion.

Repeat steps 1–3.

4

Using the flat of your hands, circle over your partner's lower back area at the base of the spine using one hand after the other, you can even rock the pelvis gently from side to side with the motion, which will feel very comforting. You will need to position yourself at the side of your partner for this stroke and you might like to finish off with some flicking (see page 33) over the buttocks, followed by feathering (see page 38) and stroking to finish off.

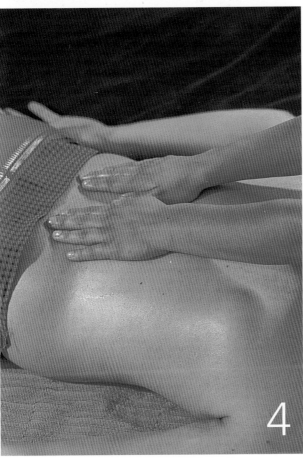

Using Sensual Massage Aids

Remember to vary your strokes for sensual massage. Use the ones that your partner prefers and do not feel inhibited or afraid to experiment – simply follow your instincts.

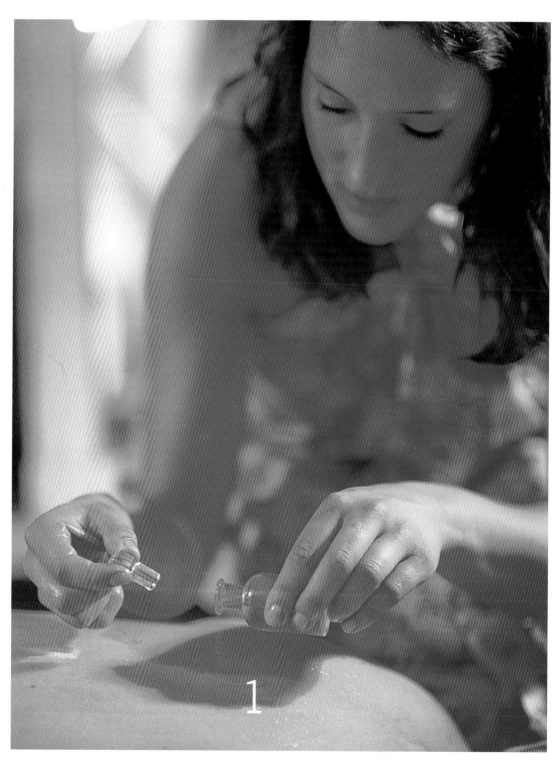

1

1

Try using diluted oils, scented with ylang ylang or jasmine, dripped directly on to the body for a different sensation.

2

Massage creams, or your favourite fragrant body lotions, are sensuous to use and will moisturize the skin at the same time, or you may prefer a powder which can be fun to use.

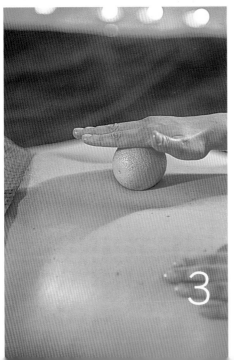

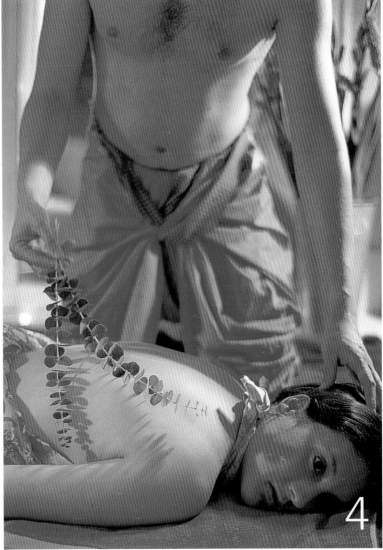

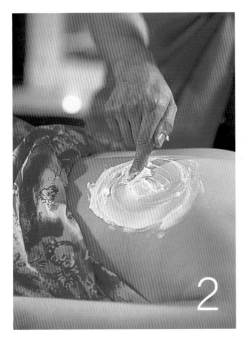

3

This is an ideal opportunity to use some massage aids (see page 40–1), as the back is a large area on which to work and is well supported. Try rolling an orange or grapefruit under your hand – as well as providing massage, the aroma of the orange soothes and warms while the grapefruit is uplifting and balancing. Alternatively, you may have a favourite massager of your own to use in this area.

4

Besides wonderful-smelling oils (as in step 1), try peacock feathers, flowers or eucalyptus, which is known for its healing properties in the winter season.

Index

Acknowledgements

Photographer Gareth Sambidge
Stylist Clare Hunt

Models
Philomena Roullard
Andrew Yhannakou / Ugly Models
Nicole Uprichard
Robert Clarke
Debbie B at Model Plan
Nicky Ross
Lucy Moore
baby Oliver Dowling

Executive Editor Jane McIntosh
Editor Abi Rowsell
Senior Designer Rozelle Bentheim
Designer Emily Wilkinson

Production Controller Viv Cracknell
Picture Researcher Jennifer Veall

A big thank you to the wonderful team at Hamlyn,
the photographer Gareth and my stars Nicola, Nikki, Lucy, Oliver, Philomena and Robbie
who brought the book to life.
On a personal note I would like to dedicate this book to all my family
and friends who have always supported me through life, my colleagues at LCM
from whom I have learnt so much and Carl for being patient with me during
the writing of this.